AF740558

# AI Augmented ECG Technology

Kang-Yin Chen • Tong Liu • Hua-Yue Tao
Editors

# AI Augmented ECG Technology

Springer

*Editors*
Kang-Yin Chen
Department of Cardiology
Second Hospital of Tianjin Medical Univ
Tianjin, China

Hua-Yue Tao
Network Information Center
Second Hospital of Tianjin Medical
University
Tianjin, China

Tong Liu
Department of Cardiology
Second Hospital of Tianjin Medical
University
President of Tianjin Institute of Cardiology
Tianjin, China

ISBN 978-981-97-8358-8 ISBN 978-981-97-8359-5 (eBook)
https://doi.org/10.1007/978-981-97-8359-5

© Tianjin Science & Technology Translation & Publishing Co., Ltd. 2024

Jointly published with Tianjin Science & Technology Translation & Publishing Co., Ltd.
The print edition is not for sale in China (Mainland). Customers from China (Mainland) please order the print book from: Tianjin Science & Technology Translation & Publishing Co., Ltd..
This work is subject to copyright. All rights are solely and exclusively licensed by the Publisher, whether the whole or part of the material is concerned, specifically the rights of reprinting, reuse of illustrations, recitation, broadcasting, reproduction on microfilms or in any other physical way, and transmission or information storage and retrieval, electronic adaptation, computer software, or by similar or dissimilar methodology now known or hereafter developed.
The use of general descriptive names, registered names, trademarks, service marks, etc. in this publication does not imply, even in the absence of a specific statement, that such names are exempt from the relevant protective laws and regulations and therefore free for general use.
The publishers, the authors, and the editors are safe to assume that the advice and information in this book are believed to be true and accurate at the date of publication. Neither the publishers nor the authors or the editors give a warranty, express or implied, with respect to the material contained herein or for any errors or omissions that may have been made. The publishers remain neutral with regard to jurisdictional claims in published maps and institutional affiliations.

This Springer imprint is published by the registered company Springer Nature Singapore Pte Ltd.
The registered company address is: 152 Beach Road, #21-01/04 Gateway East, Singapore 189721, Singapore

If disposing of this product, please recycle the paper.

# Contents

# About the Editors

**Kang-Yin Chen, MD, PhD** Chief Physician, Doctoral Supervisor, and Vice President of the Second Hospital of Tianjin Medical University. In recent years, he has devoted himself to clinical research in interventional cardiology and the application of AI technology in cardiovascular diseases.

**Hua-Yue Tao** Master of Management, Senior Engineer, Master Supervisor, and Director of the Network Information Center of the Second Hospital of Tianjin Medical University. He has long been committed to research in the field of medical informatization and the application of Internet technology and AI technology in the medical field.

**Tong Liu, MD, PhD, FESC, FHRS** Doctoral Supervisor, Director of the Department of Cardiology, Second Hospital of Tianjin Medical University, and President of Tianjin Institute of Cardiology. He is mainly engaged in basic and clinical research on atrial fibrillation and cardio-oncology.

# Overview of AI

# 1

Hua-Yue Tao, Kang-Yin Chen, Zhen Wan, Qin Xu,
Xiao-Dong Shi, and Bao-Shuai Zhang

## 1.1 Fundamentals of Artificial Intelligence

Hua-Yue Tao

In recent years, artificial intelligence (AI) has emerged as a powerful catalyst for driving social and economic progress, assuming a pivotal role in enhancing productivity, facilitating socio-economic growth, and catalyzing economic transformations. The Fifth World Intelligence Congress in 2021 showed us a future with fresh advancements in scientific exploration and charted a novel trajectory for the intelligent industry. Propelled by the advancements in big data technology, AI has been experiencing a dynamic surge, which is radically reshaping our daily existence, steering the course of China's economic evolution, and setting an unprecedented pace and scope for future developments.

The origins of AI trace back to its inception in 1956, and over the ensuing half-century, particularly in the last decade, it has embarked on an epoch of rapid acceleration. The synergistic force of "Internet Plus," "cloud computing," "big data," and "AI" has spearheaded a transformative wave of technological innovation. "Internet Plus" orchestrates the fusion of information and Internet platforms with

H.-Y. Tao (✉) · K.-Y. Chen · B.-S. Zhang
The Second Hospital of Tianjin Medical University, Tianjin, China
e-mail: zhangbaoshuai@tmu.edu.cn

Z. Wan
Haihe Hospital, Tianjin University, Tianjin, China

Q. Xu
College of Intelligence and Computing, Tianjin University, Tianjin, China
e-mail: qingxu@tju.edu.cn

X.-D. Shi
Tianjin Dafangzhongbang Computer Science and Technology Co., Ltd, Tianjin, China

© The Author(s), under exclusive license to Springer Nature Singapore Pte Ltd. 2024

K.-Y. Chen et al. (eds.), *AI Augmented ECG Technology*,
https://doi.org/10.1007/978-981-97-8359-5_1

conventional industries, refining the economic paradigm of traditional sectors. The dawn of the "cloud computing" and "big data" eras contributes a treasure trove of data assets to nourish AI development, enabling the exploration of more sophisticated algorithmic models. Meanwhile, the advent of "AI" heralds the emergence of novel products, industries, and paradigms, triggering substantial shifts in the economic framework, fundamentally altering human production, lifestyle, cognition, and fostering a comprehensive leap in societal productivity.

Despite the increasing integration of AI technology across diverse facets of human existence, a fundamental question arises: what exactly is AI? AI constitutes a novel domain of technical science that delves into the exploration and advancement of theories, methodologies, technologies, and application frameworks aimed at emulating, extending, and amplifying human intelligence. Situated within the realm of computer science, AI is the study focusing on the utilization of computational capabilities to replicate certain cognitive processes and intelligent behaviors, such as learning, reasoning, thinking, and planning. This discipline predominantly revolves around empowering computers with the ability to attain intellectuality and develop cognitive prowess akin to the human brain, thereby enabling computers to achieve elevated levels of functionality and utility.

AI exhibits the following distinct attributes.

### 1.1.1 Provide Services to Humanity Through Computational Processes and Data Manipulation

Fundamentally rooted in computation and data analysis, AI operates on the premise of being human-centric. These systems, crafted by human ingenuity, operate in accordance with program logic and software algorithms defined by human, facilitated by hardware components like microchips conceived by human. The essence of AI resides in its computational nature. Its fundamental purpose is to provide services that augment human capacities, simulating certain "intelligent behaviors" that align with human expectations. In an ideal context, these services must align with human-centric traits, safeguarding against harm to individuals and refraining from any purposeful engagement in actions detrimental to human.

### 1.1.2 Enhance External Perception and Human Interaction

AI is equipped to perceive and engage with the external environment, serving to complement human interactions. AI systems possess the capability to utilize sensors and similar devices, enabling them to sense the surrounding environment, including human presence. Like human, AI can gather information from the environment through senses such as hearing, vision, smell, and touch. It is capable of generating text, speech, expressions, actions (control mechanisms), and other pertinent responses to external inputs, thereby influencing the environment or human interactions. By means of buttons, keyboards, screens, gestures, expressions, force feedback, and virtual/augmented reality, human can effectively communicate and collaborate with machines, and, in the meanwhile, machines can have a better "understanding" of what human want them to do, thereby fostering collaboration and mutual support. In this symbiotic relationship, AI can undertake tasks that might not align with human preferences or expertise but are well-suited for machine execution. Meanwhile, human can focus on tasks demanding creativity, insight, imagination, adaptability, variability, and even emotional understanding, thereby optimizing the division of labor.

### 1.1.3 The Capability of Adapting, Learning, Evolving, and Iterating

In an ideal context, an AI system should exhibit adaptive qualities and a learning capability. This implies that the system should be able to dynamically adjust parameters or update optimization models in response to changes in the environment, data, or tasks. Furthermore, leveraging extensive and deep digital connections with the cloud, individuals, and objects enables the evolution and iteration of both machine entities and even human subjects. This enhances the system's adaptability, robustness, flexibility, and scalability, enabling it to effectively navigate the ever-shifting real-world environment and generate diverse applications across various domains.

In essence, the domain of AI primarily revolves around imbuing machines with the ability to perceive, acquire knowledge, store information, reason, think, learn, and execute actions, among other human-like attributes. The ultimate goal is to create intelligent systems that mimic human cognition or transcend it. Currently, computers serve as the principal tools for studying and realizing AI technology. The evolution of AI is intertwined with the progress of computer science and technology. AI research spans various fields, including computer science, neuroscience, psychology, linguistics, logic, cognitive science, behavior science, as well as mathematics, information theory, cybernetics, and system theory.

The key focal points of AI research encompass knowledge representation, automated reasoning, search methodologies, machine learning (ML), and knowledge acquisition. Other crucial areas include knowledge processing systems, natural language comprehension, computer vision, intelligent robotics, and automated programming.

## 1.2 AI's Impact on the Medical Domain

Hua-Yue Tao and Kang-Yin Chen

The applications of AI technology within the medical sector are diverse, encompassing various stages of medical procedures such as pre-hospital management, in-hospital diagnosis and treatment, and post-hospital rehabilitation. This integration has found utility across multiple domains within clinical medicine. The synergy between AI and the medical field predominantly relies on machine learning algorithms and big data analytics. Leveraging AI technology brings forth improved medical service efficiency, reduces comprehensive service costs, and catalyzes the overall advancement of the medical domain.

Recent years have seen the establishment of hospital-level, regional, and national medical data centers, largely propelled by pertinent national policies. As medical clinical big data attains greater refinement and standardization, its applications extend into specialized realms, culminating in the emergence of a medical big data industry. AI and big data technologies operate by formulating intricate rules within extensive data repositories. This entails the extraction of pertinent information for reclassification and integration. By merging medical knowledge maps with clinical diagnostic and treatment experiences, machine deep learning (DL) emulates human diagnosis and treatment processes, generating clinically relevant insights.

The integration of AI technology into medical diagnosis mandates rigorous professional validation to ensure heightened reliability and accuracy. Ultimately, this paves the way for the creation of an intelligent diagnosis and treatment system founded on AI technology. The concurrent development of the medical big data industry alongside AI's penetration into the medical landscape expedites the evolution of medical intelligence. This synergy lays a robust scientific foundation for AI-based diagnosis and auxiliary clinical support.

### 1.2.1 International AI Advancements in the Medical Realm

The inception of AI's foray into the medical domain traces back to the 1970s. In 1972, a pioneering application known as AA-PHelp, developed by the University of Leeds, marked the initial stride in utilizing AI systems for medical purposes. This system primarily supported the auxiliary diagnosis of acute abdominal pain, catering to surgical requirements. Subsequently, a series of systems like INTERNISTI, MYCINCASNET/Glaucoma, PIP, and ABEL emerged, each with varying degrees of efficacy. The 1980s witnessed the emergence of commercial AI application systems, such as QMR (Quick Medical Reference) and DXplain from Harvard Medical School, which offered diagnostic schemes aligned with clinical manifestations.

Presently, a prominent figure in the medical AI landscape is IBM/Watson. This advanced system is able to sift rapidly through decades of cancer treatment history encompassing millions of patient records to swiftly furnish physicians with evidence-based alternative treatment plans. The convergence of "AI+" with medical research has recently become a focal point in modern science and technology. Renowned American medical institutions, including Mayo Clinic and Cleveland Clinic, have initiated collaborations with AI companies, envisioning a future where they serve as epicenters for AI medical applications, encompassing disease detection, diagnosis, treatment, and management. Currently, AI has assumed a significant role across diverse dimensions of the medical landscape, encompassing areas like medical image recognition, biotechnology, and supplementary functions. Among these, medical image recognition stands out as a prevalent application, especially in realms such as diagnosis, drug R&D, and nutrition. Looking ahead, the role of AI in the medical arena is poised to undergo further transformation, potentially revolutionizing medical approaches and even the very paradigms of healthcare. This transformation holds the potential to catalyze advancements in the medical field, reshape the structure of the medical industry, and even influence the future trajectories of certain medical practitioners. It is firmly believed that AI's impending influence will usher in profound shifts in future medical technologies, serving as a formidable catalyst for innovation and comprehensive reform within the healthcare sector.

### 1.2.2 Present Domestic Development Landscape

In terms of national influence, the top five countries spearheading AI advancements are the United States, China, the United Kingdom, Canada, and India. Notably, China leads with the highest proportion of AI applications in the medical and health sector, accounting for a substantial 22%. Recent years have witnessed China issuing a series of pivotal policy documents focusing on medical AI. "Made in China 2025," a directive released by the State Council in May 2015, places a strategic emphasis on advancing high-performance diagnostic and treatment equipment like imaging apparatus and medical robots. In May 2016, the *"Internet Plus" Artificial Intelligence Three-Year Action and Implementation Plan* outlined critical projects encompassing intelligent wearable devices, intelligent robotic R&D, and applications. This initiative fostered the growth and implementation of AI within the medical domain. In June 2016, the General Office of the State Council issued the *Guiding Opinions on Promoting and Regulating the Application and Development of Big Data in Healthcare* recognizing healthcare data's role as a vital strategic resource with the potential to substantially transform the healthcare model. In July 2017, the State Council released the *Development Plan for the New Generation of Artificial Intelligence*, delineating the trajectories for smart medicine evolution. This roadmap encompassed constructs like smart hospitals, surgical robots, intelligent diagnosis, physiological monitoring, image recognition, new drug R&D, pharmaceutical oversight, and intelligent epidemic monitoring and prevention. Bolstered by diverse policy support, medical AI in China has achieved commendable milestones across multiple domains. For instance, in the realm of clinical medical intelligent decision-making, collaborative efforts between Beijing Yasen Technology Development Co., Ltd. and prominent hospitals such as Beijing Xuanwu Hospital, Peking University People's Hospital, and Union Medical College Hospital have yielded remarkable results. Deployed across over 30 large-scale Grade III-A hospitals, their brain function multi-modal AI products have successfully conducted over 7000 case analyses, boasting an impressive average accuracy rate exceeding 84% for various ailments. Underpinned by the "Internet Plus" medical policy, a multitude of internet-based companies have emerged in the medical market, focusing on online consultations, expert registrations, medical e-commerce, and medical insurance. Looking ahead, China is poised to address challenges such as the uneven distribution and concentration of medical resources through internet-driven solutions. Currently, research in the medical and health AI arena is becoming increasingly sophisticated, exerting a profound influence on the trajectory of medical and healthcare development.

## 1.3 Application Basis of AI Technology in the Realm of ECG Diagnosis

Zhen Wan and Hua-Yue Tao

### 1.3.1 Leveraging Big Data Analytics

AI relies heavily on the processing of vast datasets, employing sophisticated algorithms to achieve its objectives. A pivotal facet of AI lies in data mining technology, where computers dissect data to generate human-centric recommendations and predictions. The realm of medical innovation holds immense potential for AI, promising substantial societal and economic benefits. The bedrock of AI's success in medical innovation rests upon the availability of digital medical big data. As medical information technology rapidly evolves, hospitals are increasingly enhancing their informatization initiatives, leading to an accumulation of substantial medical data within the healthcare sector. In this era marked by an exponential surge in data, exhaustive analysis of massive datasets can identify challenges and offer viable solutions.

Presently, hospitals are grappling with fragmented medical data management systems. A proliferation of diverse and uncoordinated hospital business management systems has resulted in copious but dispersed data. The current state of affairs lacks comprehensive data content, thwarting data sharing between various information systems. The absence of a unified standard display platform further constrains information utilization, impeding user searches and the formulation of effective decision support mechanisms.

### 1.3.2 Progressing Through Stages of Big Data Analysis

With the ongoing progression of informatization, the maturity of data analysis and data mining technologies for medical big data becomes increasingly apparent. Data processing can be segmented into four distinctive stages.

#### 1.3.2.1 Data Extraction

The initial stage involves extracting target data from the source system. This process includes data source group management, application model construction, and the extraction of essential data fields.

#### 1.3.2.2 Data Integration

Data integration encompasses the synthesis and aggregation of disparate datasets, resolving the fusion and association of diverse data types. Through the establishment of primary indices and adhering to specific standards, data can be analyzed for their comprehensive correlation. Multi-source heterogeneous data is integrated, thereby fostering data standardization and facilitating the creation of clinical data centers. This framework, comprising a standard system and traceability system, proficiently manages multi-source heterogeneous data.

#### 1.3.2.3 Data Storage

Employing distributed big data technology, data storage entails distributed data storage methods optimized for intricate medical data. Constructing numerous distributed data computing nodes allows for multi-dimensional expression of medical data.

#### 1.3.2.4 Data Analysis

Data analysis involves the application of AI systems that utilize machine learning, natural language processing, and pattern recognition to replicate human cognitive processes. Through machine learning or deep learning algorithms, computer systems are trained to autonomously solve problems, obviating the need for human intervention.

### 1.3.3 Crucial Components of Big Data Analysis

At the heart of AI lies machine learning, serving as its fundamental bedrock. Machine learning employs algorithms to deconstruct data, learn from it, and subsequently make informed decisions and predictions regarding real-world events. In stark contrast to conventional software, machine learning is "trained" using substantial data, mastering tasks via a variety of algorithms.

#### 1.3.3.1 Natural Language Processing

Natural language processing involves computer technology analyzing, comprehending, and processing human language to generate machine-readable text.

#### 1.3.3.2 Pattern Recognition

Pattern recognition employs computational methods to categorize samples based on distinctive characteristics. This encompasses the automated processing and interpretation of patterns utilizing mathematical techniques.

As the integration of AI with medical treatment deepens, AI-assisted technologies have permeated various medical domains. Electrocardiogram (ECG) examination, a staple in clinical medicine, captures changes in heart electrical activity via surface recordings, serving as a pivotal tool in diagnosing ailments such as arrhythmia, myocardial ischemia, myocardial infarction, and cardiac enlargement. ECG data, a vital subset of medical information, is central to ECG big data, with accurate interpretation serving as its core. While software-driven ECG analysis is indispensable in clinical practice, its efficacy remains insufficient to supplant manual interpretation. Leveraging big data analysis holds the potential to minimize manual intervention, enhance automatic analysis accuracy, and transform cardiovascular disease diagnosis. The integration of AI systems bolsters precise cardiovascular disease diagnosis, enabling quantitative health prediction and early health management. The amalgamation of machine learning, data cleaning, distributed storage, and data mining augments data integration, facilitating the evolution of scattered data into a knowledge repository conducive to machine learning. By immersing in the analysis of extensive ECG data, software systems can progressively "learn" ECG interpretation through historical data assimilation and ongoing optimization. This dynamic culminates in an application model primed for ECG interpretation. Ongoing research in data analysis and machine learning is poised to render significant contributions to individual health, diagnostic support, public health, and beyond.

## 1.4 AI-Powered ECG Interpretation Methods

Xu Qing and Hua-Yue Tao

ECGs have long been instrumental in unveiling insights into both cardiac and non-cardiac health conditions, yet deciphering the intricate information they encapsulate demands substantial expertise and experience. Modern AI technology, spearheaded by deep learning, stands poised to swiftly emulate human-like ECG interpretation, extending its aid not only to medical professionals but also to non-specialists. The original ECG data are primarily presented in graphical and structured formats. Guided by task-specific feature extraction, neural networks are fed with ECG data and meticulously fine-tuned for analysis. When confronted with raw ECG data, deep learning neural networks adeptly dissect the intricate data structure, identify vital features, undertake targeted classification tasks, and culminate in comprehensive data interpretation. The successful utilization of deep learning neural networks in ECG analysis has particularly excelled in accurate identification of arrhythmias (with a pronounced focus on atrial fibrillation and normal sinus rhythm), cardiac insufficiency, electrolyte imbalances, sleep apnea, and related symptoms. Notably, convolutional neural networks (CNNs), recurrent neural networks (RNNs), deep neural networks (DNNs), and hybrid models comprising multiple networks have gained widespread prominence as effective network architectures [1, 2]. The process of interpreting ECG data through deep learning neural networks chiefly involves three pivotal steps: data preprocessing, feature extraction, and classification. Data preprocessing encompasses vital operations such as band-pass filtering, discrete wavelet transform, short-time Fourier transform, and normalization. These operations collectively diminish noise and interference, rendering the data more amenable to feature extraction and neural network training. Feature extraction entails techniques such as convolution, pooling, and correction, uncovering salient attributes within the ECG data. Subsequently, classification strives to categorize disparate features based on the identified attributes, adapting relevant interpretations and iteratively optimizing neural network parameters via backpropagation.

The ensuing examples illustrate diverse deep learning neural network models and their distinctive processing methodologies for ECG data, whether presented in graphical or structured formats.

### 1.4.1 Graphical Comparative Approach

When ECG data is represented graphically, the paramount objective is to extract spatial features inherent in the graph. This methodology involves a series of steps: initially, effective segments within the ECG are isolated through techniques such as graph recombination, Fourier transform, and wavelet scale transform. These selected segments are then input into a neural network model to generate feature maps. By discerning distinctions among various features and correlating them with pertinent medical interpretations, this process culminates in output judgments during practical testing. These judgments support both medical professionals and non-specialists in the interpretation of ECG data.

CNN: Attia et al. [3] harnessed a dataset of 35,970 paired ECGs (comprising standard 10-s 12-lead ECGs) along with contemporaneous transthoracic echocardiograms to introduce a groundbreaking CNN-based screening technique. This innovation aimed to identify patients with reduced left ventricular function (ejection fraction ≤35%). Evaluated on a dataset of 52,870 ECGs, this network model demonstrated impressive metrics, including an area under the curve (AUC) of 0.93, sensitivity of 86.3%, specificity of 85.7%, and an overall accuracy of 85.7%.

DNN: Hannun et al. [4] devised a pioneering end-to-end deep learning method for ECG interpretation, undertaking a comprehensive evaluation across an array of common ECG rhythm categories. These categories encompassed atrial fibrillation/flutter, atrioventricular block, great artery systole, ectopic atrial rhythm, ventricular autonomic rhythm, junctional rhythm, noise, sinus rhythm, supraventricular tachycardia, tricuspid valve, ventricular tachycardia, and Vencil-type conduction. The study employed a single-lead, mount-based mobile ECG monitoring device to gather a vast dataset of 91,232 single-lead ECGs from 53,549 patients to train their DNN model. The architecture of this neural network comprised 34 layers, incorporating 16 residual blocks, each housing 2 convolutional layers. Upon assessment with an independent test dataset, the DNN model achieved an impressive average ROC AUC of 0.97. Notably, the DNN model's sensitivity surpassed the average sensitivity achieved by expert cardiologists while maintaining comparable specificity levels.

### 1.4.2 Structured Data Comparative Approach

In contrast to the graphical representation of ECG data, employing deep neural networks with structured data primarily centers on extracting relational features among the data, such as the temporal evolution of ECG signals. This approach often involves displaying structured ECG data as one- or two-dimensional arrays. After undergoing preprocessing steps including normalization, segmentation, and filtering, the array's numerical attributes—such as time, frequency, and amplitude—are extracted through neural network-based techniques. These attributes, highlighting disparities, are subsequently categorized. Throughout this interpretation process, ECG insights are provided to both medical practitioners and individuals without specialized training.

RNN: Zhou et al. [5] introduced a method utilizing long short-term memory (LSTM) within a RNN framework to facilitate arrhythmia classification. Their model initially utilizes wavelet basis functions to eliminate external artifact influence within the two-dimensional ECG signal data. By determining segment lengths within the signal and segmenting R-R interval data, the model proceeds to standardize the data through dominant transformation. Subsequently, the LSTM network extracts interval, duration, and amplitude parameters from the ECG signal's time domain, facilitating arrhythmia classification based on distinctive characteristics. Through comprehensive independent testing and evaluation, the proposed network model displayed superior performance compared to other AI methodologies.

Hybrid Models: Kwon et al. [6] devised an innovative model for diagnosing left ventricular hypertrophy by merging CNN and DNN components. Their approach involved generating 12 × 4000 2D data from each 10-s ECG recording encompassing 12 leads, augmented with demographic details (age, gender, weight, and height). CNN and DNN structures were combined, involving convolution, pooling, flattening, and batch normalization steps. These processes extracted diagnostic features for identifying left ventricular hypertrophy symptoms, visibly displayed through visualization technology on critical ECG segments. The hybrid network model achieved an impressive AUC of 0.868, with the sensitivity of the ensemble neural network (ENN) at 0.432, exceeding the average sensitivity of cardiologists' assessments by 152.1%, all while maintaining comparable specificity (0.951).

## 1.5 Implementation of Remote ECG Consultation System Via Mobile Terminals and Clinical Big Data

Shi Xiaodong, Hua-Yue Tao, and Zhang Baoshuai

As the Internet era advances at breakneck speed, the pivotal role of big data within the medical and healthcare sectors has garnered escalating attention. This has catalyzed a gradual shift from the traditional medical paradigm to an increasingly mobile medical model. In 2017, governmental initiatives embarked on promoting the establishment of "medical alliances" with the overarching goal of orchestrating the integration of regional medical resources. The purpose of these alliances is to bridge high-quality medical resources vertically and horizontally, thereby enhancing primary medical services, refining the medical service system, and fostering the creation of a coherent and structured hierarchical diagnosis and treatment framework [7–8].

However, the rapid evolution of the medical consortium model has also brought to the forefront certain undeniable challenges, most notably the issue of "interconnectivity deficiency" [9]. Various medical institutions, particularly those spanning different tiers, have struggled to establish a seamless information-sharing mechanism. The lack of interconnectedness has led to fragmented residents' health data, disjointed patient medical records, and non-recognition of examination and test outcomes. These disparities resulted in escalated medical expenses and even heightened risks of delayed diagnoses or misdiagnoses.

Furthermore, primary health service establishments often grapple with an insufficiency of adept personnel. Medical practitioners with limited education, inadequate professional skills, and service proficiency find it challenging to meet the rigorous demands of higher-tier hospitals for referrals. Conversely, physicians in Grade III-A hospitals contend with hectic schedules, hampering their ability to dedicate substantial time to consultation sessions. This predicament particularly hampers the bidirectional referral process essential for effective management of chronic conditions, ultimately impeding the seamless implementation of hierarchical diagnosis and treatment frameworks.

Hence, the need of the hour is to urgently establish a comprehensive big data platform rooted in mobile terminal technology, facilitating seamless information sharing and fostering real-time interaction. This robust infrastructure holds the potential to revolutionize the landscape of remote ECG consultation, surmounting prevailing challenges and ushering in a new era of enhanced medical collaboration and holistic patient care. In line with our objectives, we proudly introduce the "Whole-Heart Linkage" initiative, a comprehensive endeavor underpinned by four fundamental principles: whole-process management, chronic disease care for heart and cardiovascular ailments, seamless connectivity, and real-time dynamism. Our overarching goal is to facilitate a holistic approach to cardiovascular disease management. As we delve into the project's conceptual framework and implementation strategy, let's explore the design ideas and comprehensive plan in detail.

### 1.5.1 Platform Planning

#### 1.5.1.1 System Evaluation

(1) Construction Objectives: In alignment with national strategies like hierarchical diagnosis and treatment, Internet-enabled healthcare, and precision medicine, our endeavor aims to establish a clinical big data research platform. This platform will facilitate chronic disease management and research by offering data support. Additionally, it will enable seamless sharing of patients' medical information, examination results, and laboratory findings between healthcare institutions. The focus is on patient-centric integration of diagnosis and treatment processes, compiling comprehensive patient records for optimized utilization of diagnostic and

treatment data. Ultimately, the platform will provide patients with extended data tracking and personalized healthcare services [10–11].

(2) Working Methods: Extensive research encompassing chronic disease management, mobile medical practices, and health-related big data has fostered the platform's design. Consultations with experts spanning diverse fields, including hospital management, clinical medicine, information engineering, big data processing, and AI, have shaped the project's goals, steps, and specifics. Integrating expert insights and recent global research findings, the platform centers on an ECG database as its core. It facilitates real-time sharing of chronic disease management data via mobile phones or tablets, forming a comprehensive big data platform (Fig. 1.1).

#### 1.5.1.2 Platform Architecture

(1) Hardware Architecture: The remote ECG consultation system's hardware components encompass ECG data acquisition equipment, terminal APP running devices, terminal PCs, and central private cloud hardware (including compute servers, storage devices, and necessary network access and management equipment). ECG data from patients is collected by doctors using ECG data acquisition equipment and terminal devices. This data is then transmitted to the central private cloud platform

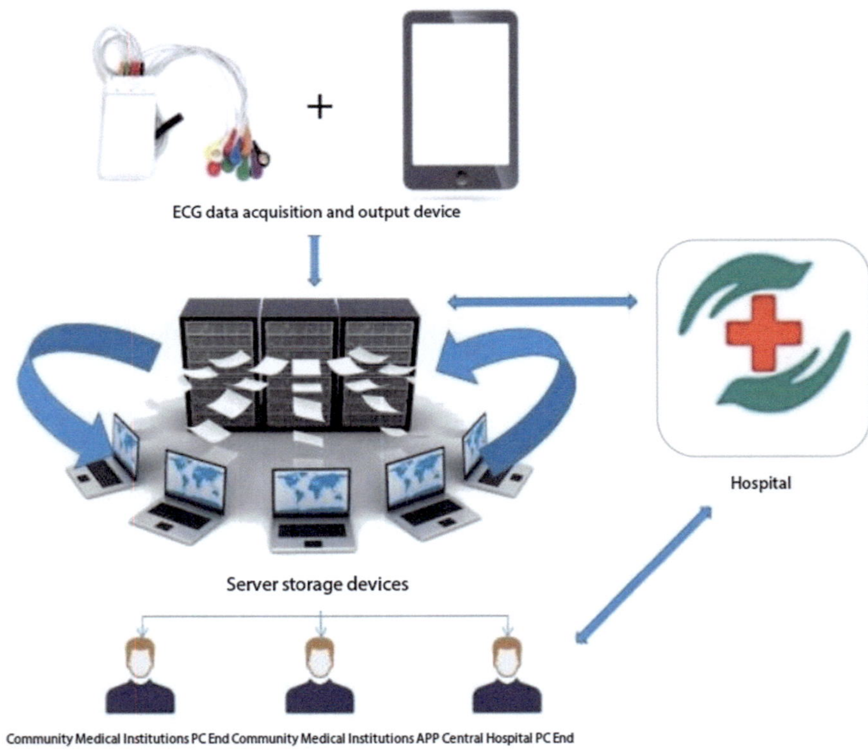


**Fig. 1.1** Remote ECG consultation network system

using wireless, wired, or internet-based technology. The central cloud platform archives and stores the data, priming it for subsequent processing. The central terminal further sends the data to the doctor's terminal device or PC for real-time viewing and diagnosis of ECG information (Fig. 1.1).

In the contemporary age of advanced Internet devices, diverse terminals (mobile phones, tablets, and computers) can serve as tools for central hospital doctors to access, view, compare, download, and print ECG image data. This versatility significantly facilitates clinicians during diagnosis and treatment [12].

Furthermore, the ECG consultation system boasts the capability to seamlessly integrate and exchange data with the central hospital's internal information systems. These include the hospital management information system (HIS), laboratory information system (LIS), picture archiving and communication system (PACS), electronic medical record (EMR), and more. This integration facilitates data sharing and establishes a robust and interconnected hospital information platform [13]. With the steadfast support of the central private cloud platform, every patient's ECG data from outpatient, emergency, and ward departments can be collected, recorded, diagnosed, stored, and transmitted across the network, thereby achieving comprehensive data sharing.

(2) Software Architecture: The remote ECG consultation system boasts an array of functionalities within its software architecture, including system interfaces, data archiving, and more. Specific features include ECG data submission, ECG report submission, ECG file retrieval, ECG data archiving, and retrieval of patient hospitalization, outpatient, and emergency information. Coupled with the extensive capabilities of the big data analysis platform, this amalgamation results in the realization of a chronic disease management big data platform. At the core of this platform lies the storage and sharing of ECG data, thereby empowering comprehensive management and insights into chronic diseases.

The system establishes a private cloud platform at the central end, serving as a repository for ECG data and associated patient medical information, thereby offering comprehensive diagnosis and data analysis capabilities. To cater to users of various roles, the client-side entails the creation of Patient APP, Community APP, Central APP, and Central PC modules, facilitating seamless services. Moreover, this network connects medical institutions spanning diverse tiers, from Grade I to III hospitals, within the radiation area. A detailed depiction of the functional framework is depicted in Fig. 1.2.

Functioning as the epicenter, the Medical Cloud Data Center encompasses external services while concurrently orchestrating internal data coordination, organization, and synchronization. This center stores fundamental patient details, clinical and image data, medical history records, ECG application, and uploaded data. The auxiliary knowledge base data further enriches this repository. Within the central private cloud, standardized data exchange protocols and formats are embraced, coupled with a loosely coupled bus communication form. This synergy ensures efficient processing of a diverse array of data types. Additionally, a patient main index service is instituted to seamlessly consolidate disparate business data and unite data

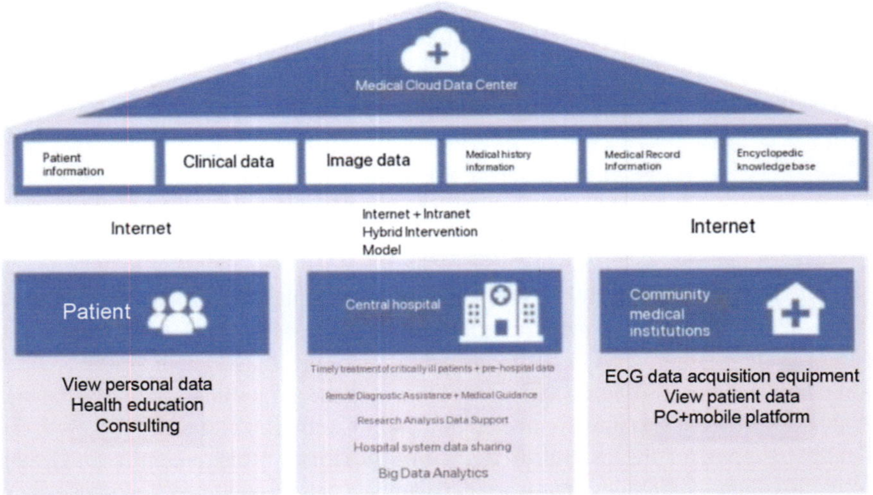


**Fig. 1.2** Functional framework of central private cloud platform

with lesser individual significance, thereby crafting comprehensive patient data units.

The user interface is thoughtfully compartmentalized into Central APP and PC Business, Lower-Level Medical Institution APP, and Patient-Centric Public APP Service, catering to the varied user demographics. The platform encompasses a wide spectrum of mobile terminal devices, accommodating users' preferences and fostering familiarity with the provided functions.

Before the commencement of ECG examinations, the system necessitates input of patient data for management, including name, hospital admission number, and ID number (medical insurance number). The system cross-references this identification information with the patient information housed within the main index service, thereby establishing a coherent record. Subsequent to the ECG examination's conclusion, the system automatically transmits ECG data to the server storage device, culminating in database storage of the ECG data.

Community hospitals initiate report applications through the mobile APP, transmitting the patient's ECG data and real-time condition to the central hospital. Experts and doctors at the central hospital can access the patient's historical medical data and diagnosis and treatment records via PC or mobile APP, subsequently issuing an ECG report based on the real-time condition. Post-report generation, the completed report is autonomously uploaded to the clinical data center, with pertinent outcomes relayed to the community hospital, which will be used as a foundational reference for ECG diagnoses. The resultant reports and image data are synchronized with the big data platform, contributing to patients' diagnostic and treatment data. Moreover, this data can be accessed for analysis and scientific research.

### 1.5.2 Implementation Results

#### 1.5.2.1 Overview of Community-Side APP Functions

The critical role of ECG in early detection and diagnosis of cardiovascular diseases is undeniable. However, interpreting ECG results requires specialized expertise, and timely and accurate diagnosis is sometimes beyond the reach of doctors in Grade I and II hospitals. Given the ongoing transition toward decentralized healthcare, a significant portion of patients receive initial diagnoses in lower-level hospitals, necessitating seamless and effective communication with higher-level medical institutions. To address this need, the remote ECG consultation system has introduced a community-side APP, empowering community doctors to upload real-time patient diagnosis and treatment information and engage in direct communication with higher-level hospital doctors (Fig. 1.3).

Upon downloading the community-side APP and logging in using their credentials, doctors gain access to the ECG consultation system. When receiving a patient, doctors navigate to the patient information interface by selecting the diagnosis and treatment application. Patient data is entered, either by inputting basic information or automatically retrieving existing records. Subsequently, doctors use data acquisition devices to collect ECG data while also having the option to verbally describe the patient's condition in an audio file or upload medical history data in photo format. Once uploaded, the ECG data is submitted to the central hospital for evaluation. The central hospital reviews the ECG information and provides treatment recommendations or referrals. Guided by these recommendations, community doctors proceed to formulate the subsequent treatment plan.

#### 1.5.2.2 Overview of Central APP Functions

Doctors access the central APP by downloading the application and logging in using their designated credentials. They can then receive patients and initiate ECG diagnoses, as facilitated by the community-side APP (Fig. 1.4).

The central APP allows doctors to diagnose ECG results and generate formal reports. By selecting the "To Report" option, doctors can view the list of patients requiring ECG reports. Selecting a patient provides access to comprehensive patient information and medical history, serving as parameters for issuing an ECG report. When composing a report, doctors can utilize pre-entered report templates, expediting the diagnostic process and enhancing efficiency. The system automatically updates the patient's inpatient and outpatient data, ensuring that doctors can quickly comprehend the patient's condition and enhancing diagnostic accuracy.

Operating in the background, the central APP generates push notifications in real-time whenever a new report is pending. Utilizing a "Didi Grab Order" model, only one doctor can access and issue a report for a specific ECG at a given time. Other doctors gain access once the initial doctor releases the ECG. This model, coupled with a suitable incentive mechanism, enhances doctor motivation and work efficiency, aligning with contemporary medical reform policies.

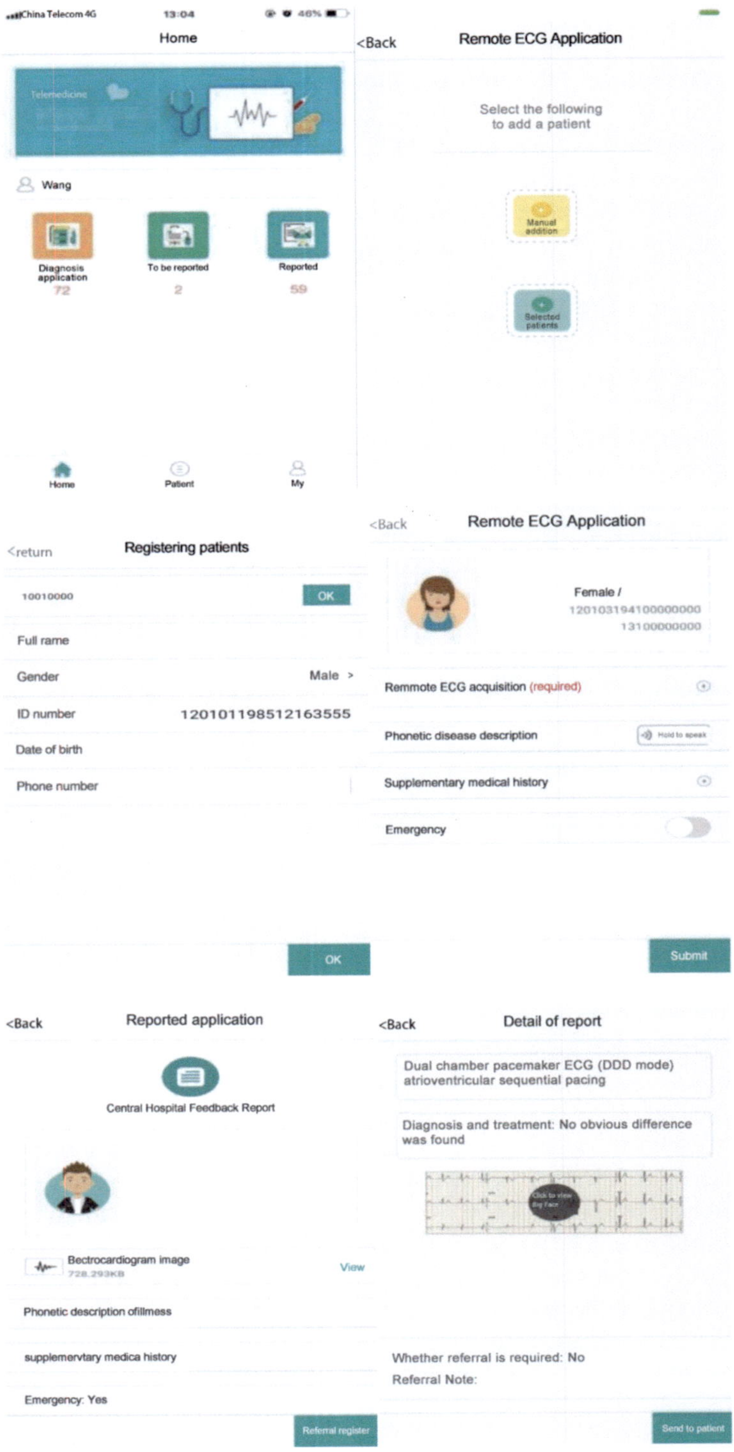


**Fig. 1.3** Community APP function snapshot

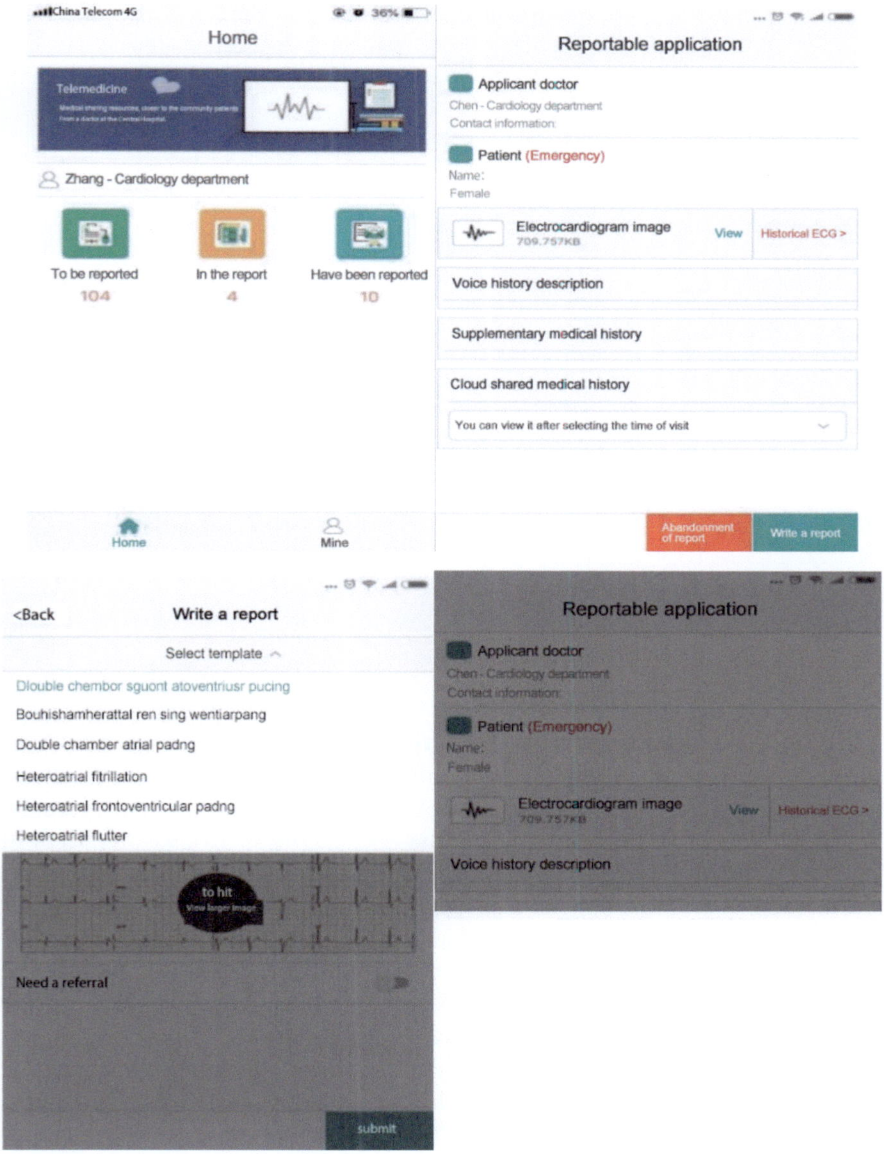


**Fig. 1.4** Center APP function snapshots

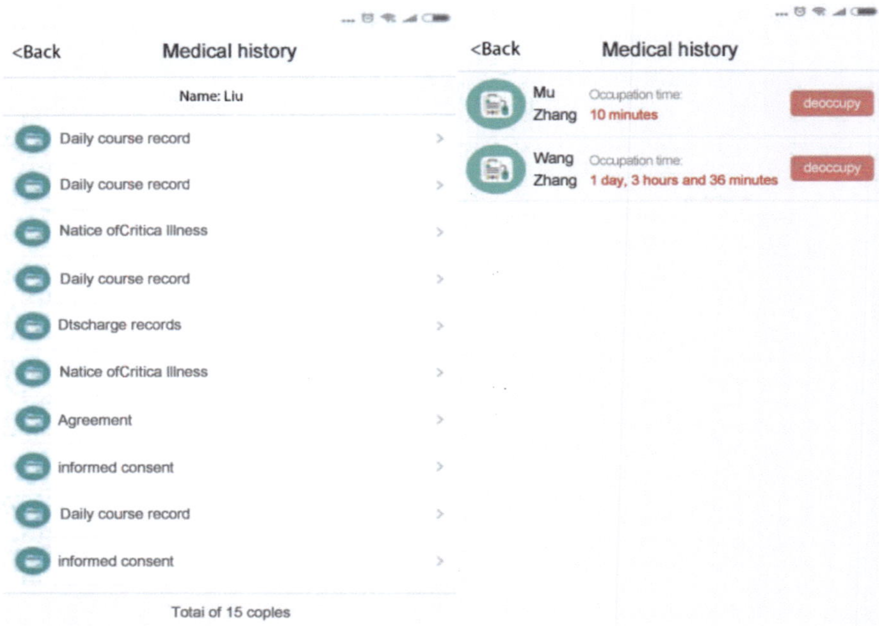


**Fig. 1.4** (continued)

#### 1.5.2.3 Overview of Central PC Terminal Functions

A central PC terminal has been thoughtfully developed for the remote ECG system, catering to specialized departments engaged in ECG information research. Within the ECG Information Center of the Second Hospital of Tianjin Medical University, an advanced multi-functional ECG analysis system is at play. ECG practitioners access this system using proprietary login credentials. This system not only facilitates ECG waveform and parameter analysis and diagnosis but also enables a comparative analysis and statistical exploration of pertinent ECG types. Furthermore, seamless data sharing and preservation are achieved between the ECG consultation system and the hospital's HIS system, PACS system, LIS system, and medical record system. These interconnected systems provide a robust foundation for the generation of precise ECG reports. The resulting ECG reports, once produced by doctors, can be promptly saved, printed, reviewed, and disseminated, thereby substantially enhancing diagnostic and treatment efficiency. Presently, the Second Hospital of Tianjin Medical University has garnered significant achievements in remote ECG monitoring, successfully establishing a comprehensive ECG monitoring and diagnosis center complete with skilled personnel and cutting-edge equipment. The adoption of the remote ECG consultation system has been extended throughout the entire hospital, progressively permeating Grade I and II hospitals within the vicinity. This progressive endeavor introduces a pioneering avenue towards medical integration and the equitable distribution of medical resources.

#### 1.5.2.4 Overview of Patient-Side APP Functions

Empowered by the comprehensive platform, the patient-side APP (Fig. 1.5) gains convenient access to their health data, allowing them to track personal physical condition trends and document routine physical sign data. These records subsequently serve as pivotal foundations for future diagnoses, effectively enhancing diagnostic accuracy and relevance. Additionally, as informed members of the public, they effortlessly acquire medical insights and consult healthcare professionals regarding their individual physical sign data, thus obtaining tailored medical and wellness guidance.

(1) Find a Doctor (Fig. 1.6). This feature facilitates efficient and precise doctor searches by allowing users to explore hospitals, doctors, departments, disease names, regions, titles, and recent browsing history for screening conditions. These functionalities expedite the process of finding the desired doctor.

(2) Interactive Consultation (Fig. 1.7). Detailed information about a doctor's expertise, practice experience, and articles can provide valuable references for patients. Patients can engage in consultations with doctors regarding specific reports or review ECG reports.

(3) ECG Report (Fig. 1.8). The ECG report list clearly distinguishes between normal and abnormal reports, allowing sorting of list content. Doctors' reports can be accessed within the report details.

(4) Physical Examination Details (Fig. 1.9). Encouraging patients to input comprehensive information about their physical examinations aids in early detection of potential diseases. This contributes to timely disease discovery, health maintenance, and cultivation of healthy lifestyle habits.

(5) Wearable Device Data Retrieval (Fig. 1.10). The Holter wearable device, capable of recording 24-h patient ECG data at home, supports data retrieval through the app.

### 1.5.3 Discussion

Analysis of practical cases reveals the intricate nature of a comprehensive Internet and chronic disease management big data platform, anchored by an ECG database as its core. This platform seamlessly integrates ECG remote diagnosis capabilities with patient clinical information. The platform achieves a standardized structure for ECG data collection, intelligently amalgamating patient ECGs, medical histories, physical signs, symptoms, and pertinent clinical data. Crucial information is extracted, serving as a comprehensive reference point for disease diagnosis and culminating in precise ECG diagnostic conclusions. The paradigm shifts away from the conventional one-dimensional diagnostic approach, commonly likened to "connecting the dots," and introduces an innovative diagnostic reference dimension. This pragmatic perspective underscores the application of AI and big data technologies, contributing to the enhancement of medical quality. As the system gains traction and wider adoption, the next phase involves establishing a research-oriented data specimen set. This facilitates deeper integration of AI technology to refine system

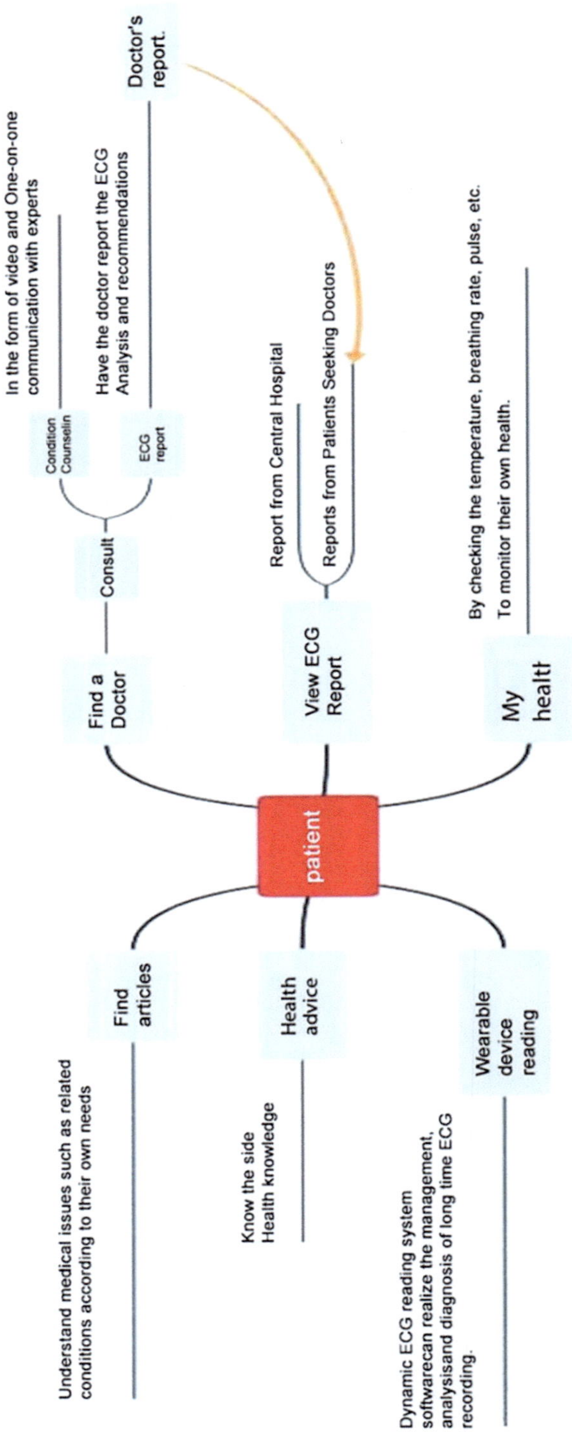


**Fig. 1.5** Patient-side APP function highlights

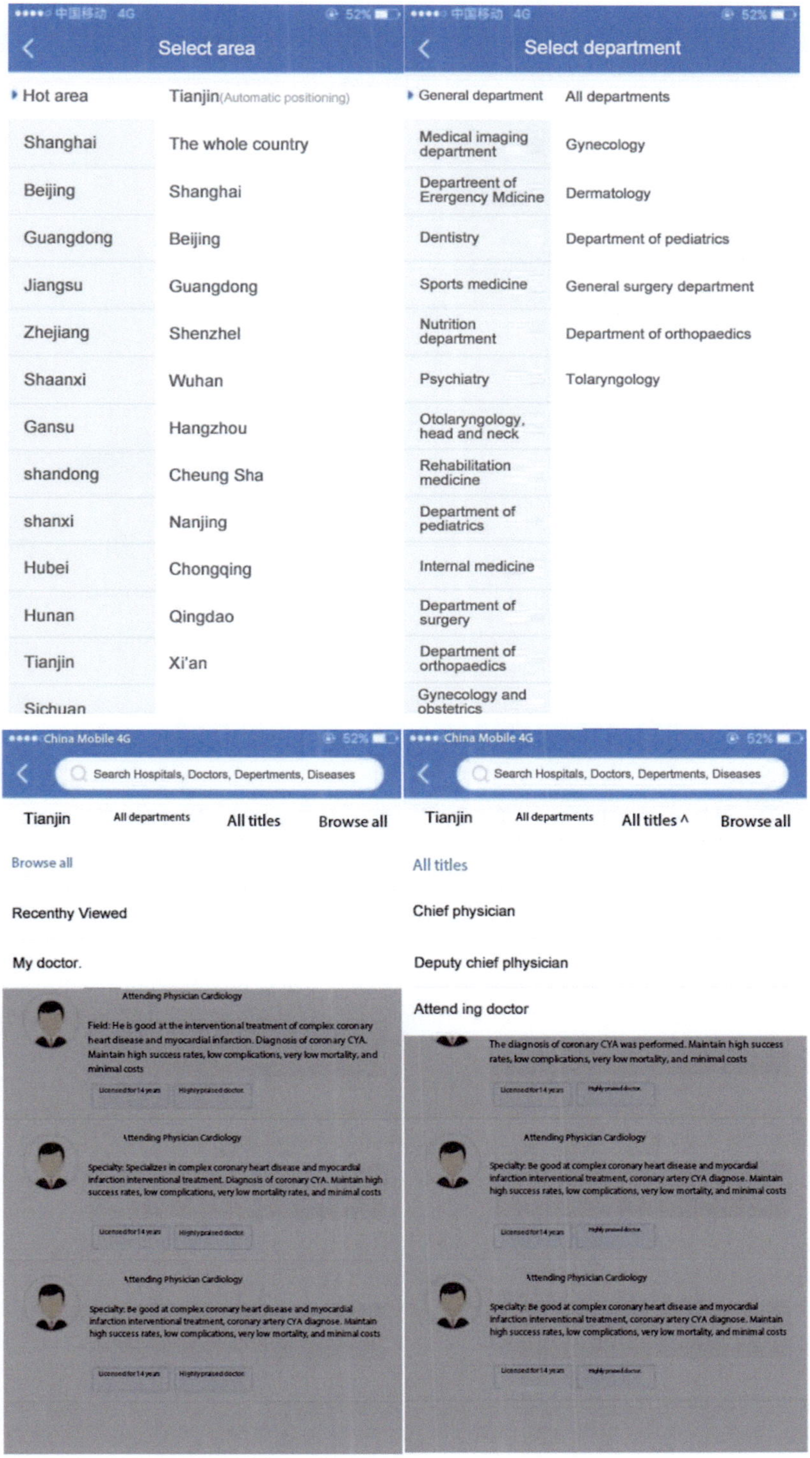


**Fig. 1.6** Patient-side APP feature—Find a doctor

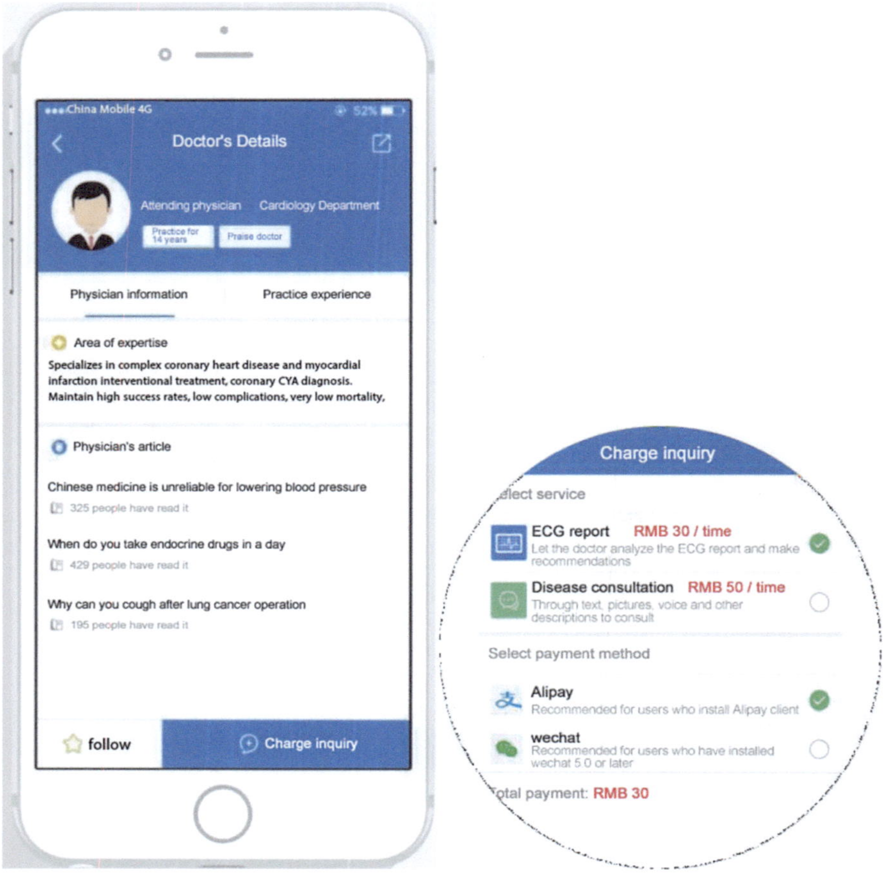


**Fig. 1.7** Patient-side APP feature—interactive consultation

AI diagnostic algorithms, thereby forming diagnostic models tailored to diverse heart-related conditions. The culmination of these efforts manifests in the tangible transformation of clinical applications through AI-powered ECG technology.

However, practical implementation has uncovered areas for further enhancement. Foremost among these is the challenge of standardizing data across the board. The pivotal role of AI technology in optimizing medical big data cannot be understated. To address this, a comprehensive expert consensus must be forged, alongside the aggregation of industry-specific data. The formulation of new standards, tailored to the AI medical realm to replace existing clinical norms, is imperative. This endeavor is further supported by the establishment of a medical data-sharing framework grounded in multi-center data aggregation. Research into data desensitization techniques and the gradual amalgamation of extensive medical databases contribute to this ongoing standardization effort. It is crucial for emerging AI technology to be intricately woven into the data standardization process, advocating for the uniformity and consistency of medical big data. This, in turn, solidifies the bedrock for successful AI applications [14].

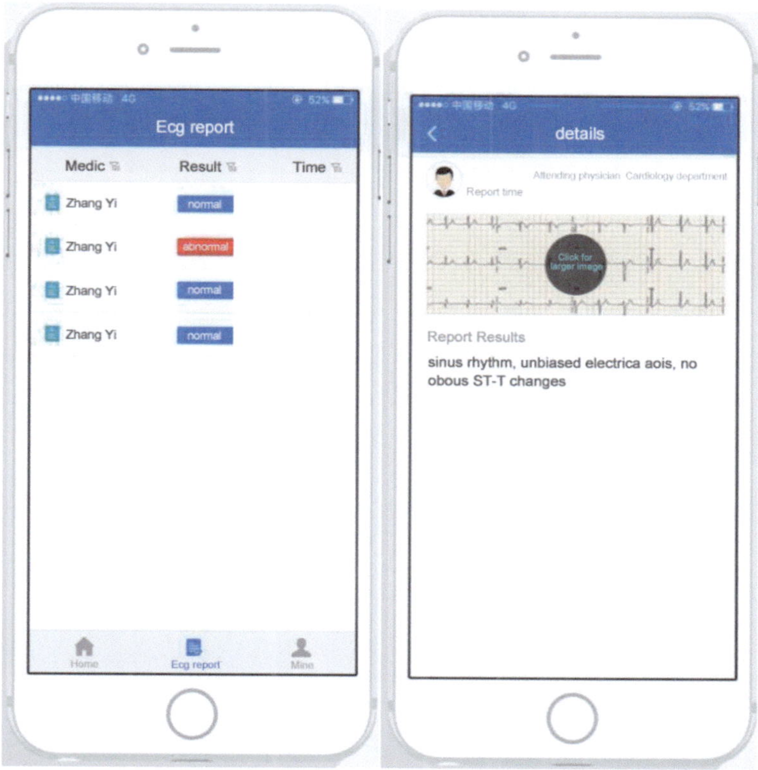


**Fig. 1.8** Patient-side APP feature—ECG report

Amid the backdrop of an all-encompassing telemedicine application framework and the active implementation of the Health China Cloud service initiative, the creation of a harmonious health and medical services integration platform, alongside the widespread adoption of computer expert consultation, augments mutual recognition and sharing mechanisms for inspection and test outcomes. This synergistic approach stimulates data resource sharing and business collaboration between major hospitals, primary medical institutions, and both developed and underdeveloped regions. The result is a fortified hierarchical diagnosis and treatment information system, firmly rooted in the Internet and big data technology. This expansion serves to magnify the service capabilities of medical and healthcare establishments, ensuring wider-reaching benefits.

Nonetheless, the human element introduces certain complexities. While AI technology is a potent tool, it mandates specialized considerations for research and implementation. In the realm of medical application, AI implementation heavily relies on machine learning, which, in turn, hinges on artificial summaries of logical laws as foundational research points for higher-level relationship learning and training. Practical experience underscores that while the platform is adept at amassing a diverse array of structured data tailored to diagnostic requirements, the journey from these data to final disease diagnosis and prediction necessitates substantial

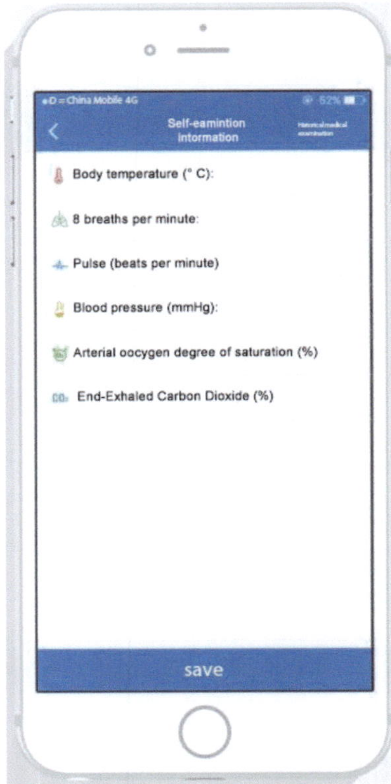


**Fig. 1.9** Patient-side APP feature—physical examination details

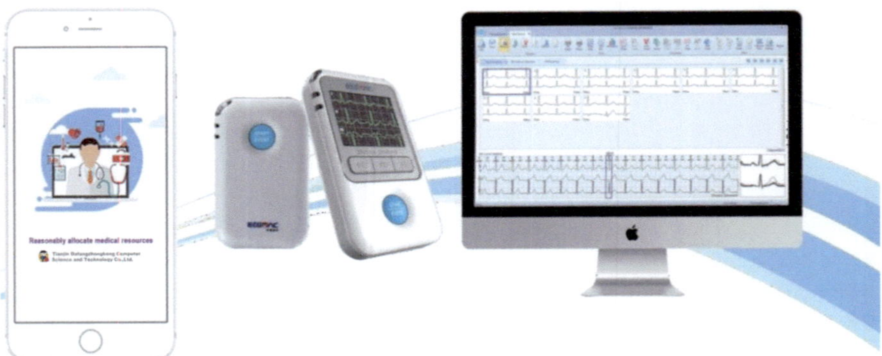

**Fig. 1.10** Patient-side APP feature—wearable device data retrieval

initial labor investment from clinical experts. These experts play an integral role in the holistic process of constructing relationships and converting prospective data into clinically significant and accurate diagnostic or predictive outcomes. In the case of intricate tasks like ECG band segmentation, a substantial corpus of medical image data, complete with precise segmentation results, is indispensable. However, the precision and volume of annotation required places significant demands on the time and energy of medical professionals. Moreover, the subjectivity inherent in annotation can impede the parameter fitting process of AI methodologies, potentially leading to inaccuracies in data-annotation mapping and subsequently affecting model performance. Notably, research into non-annotated learning methods within the realm of machine learning shows promise. This approach extracts intrinsic relationships from unlabeled data for disease phenotype classification and other investigations. However, the absence of objective and consistent criteria for evaluating research outcomes complicates the accurate assessment of performance and diminishes interpretability. As a technical tool, AI technology remains unable to entirely supplant medical experts. Given the dynamic evolution of medical knowledge and the inherent complexity of medicine itself, the development of AI systems necessitates deep involvement from medical experts [15].

In essence, the rapid progression of AI technology and its seamless integration with the medical domain are catalyzing a profound shift in the traditional medical paradigm. The fusion of AI with existing Internet technologies opens a new realm of possibilities, paving the way for AI-assisted clinical diagnosis and transformative healthcare advancements.

## References


1. Lyu J. Improvement of hierarchical diagnosis and treatment system under deepening medical and health reform. Chin Hosp Manage. 2014;34(6):1–3.
2. Ying ZX, Zeng HA, Yang QS, et al. Thinking of good quality medical resources Issues of large urban hospitals sinking to the county. Chinese Hosp Manage. 2013;33(6):1–3.
3. Tian HR, Zhang ZP. Analysis of difficulties in implementing two-way referral between hospital and community health service institutions. Clin Ration Drug Use. 2011;4(1):110.
4. Liu M, Yin YC. Research on the construction of hospital informatization connotation. J Med Inf. 2010;31:10–3.
5. Liu YQ, Chen YD. To explore the application of clinical large database to clinicians in scientific research and clinical practice. Scientif Time. 2015;12:25–7.
6. Liu ST, Wang YJ, Zhang XX, et al. Clinical research of ECG data transmission by cable network. Chin Med Equip J. 2014;35(9):122–23,32.
7. Gong YT, Guo LL, Wang B. Design and application of digital ECG network system. Chin Med Equip J. 2013;34(7):91–2.
8. Gao F, Thiebes S, Sunyaev A. Rethinking the meaning of cloud computing for health care: a taxonomic perspective and future research directions. J Med Internet Res. 2018;20(7):e10041.
9. Sun YC, Gao JD, Wu J. Artificial intelligence in clinical medicine: typical application and challenges. Chin J Stroke. 2021;16(07):643–8.
10. Sun JY, Shen H, Qu Q, et al. The application of deep learning in electrocardiogram: where we came from and where we should go. Int J Cardiol. 2021;337(4):71–8.
11. Hong S, Zhou Y, Shang J, et al. Opportunities and challenges of deep learning methods for electrocardiogram data: a systematic review. Comput Biol Med. 2020;122(5):103801.
12. Attia ZI, Kapa S, Lopez-Jimenez F, et al. Screening for cardiac contractile dysfunction using an artificial intelligence–enabled electrocardiogram. Nat Med. 2019;25(1):70–4.
13. Hannun AY, Rajpurkar P, Haghpanahi M, et al. Cardiologist-level arrhythmia detection and classification in ambulatory electrocardiograms using a deep neural network. Nat Med. 2019;25(1):65–9.
14. Zhou R, Li X, Yong B, et al. Arrhythmia recognition and classification through deep learning-based approach. Int J Comput Sci Eng. 2019;19(4):506–18.
15. Joon-Myoung K, Ki-Hyun J, Mee KH, et al. Comparing the performance of artificial intelligence and conventional diagnosis criteria for detecting left ventricular hypertrophy using electrocardiography. Europace. 2019;22(3):412–9.

# Evolution and Advancements in ECG Device Technology

# 2

Kang-Yin Chen and Hua-Yue Tao

## 2.1 Genesis of the ECG

Kang-Yin Chen

The inception of the ECG machine, a monumental achievement, is attributed to the pioneering efforts of Dutch physiologist Einthoven. In the year 1903, Einthoven unveiled the world's first practical ECG apparatus. His work extended further in 1908 when he formally introduced the concept of standard limb leads and Einthoven's equilateral triangle theory. These contributions not only laid the foundation for ECG theory but also established enduring principles that continue to shape ECG practice. This invention marked a paradigm shift, revolutionizing the landscape of cardiovascular disease diagnosis and treatment.

Although Einthoven's legacy is universally acknowledged as pivotal to modern electrocardiology, the goal to comprehend the electrical dynamics of the heart's muscular activity predates his work. The exploration of cardiac electrical activity commenced in 1842 when Matteucci uncovered the electrical behavior of frog hearts. Subsequently, in 1843, German physiologist Dubois-Reymond, an electrophysiology trailblazer, was the first to employ action potentials in describing cardiac muscle contractions. A significant stride transpired in 1856 as Koelliker and Muller recorded the human heart's electrical activity, laying the groundwork for the future ECG. Building on this legacy, French physiologist Marey harnessed a capillary

K.-Y. Chen (✉)
The Second Hospital of Tianjin Medical University, Tianjin, China

H.-Y. Tao
Director of Network Information Center of the Second Hospital of Tianjin Medical University, Tianjin, China

© The Author(s), under exclusive license to Springer Nature Singapore Pte Ltd. 2024
K.-Y. Chen et al. (eds.), *AI Augmented ECG Technology*,
https://doi.org/10.1007/978-981-97-8359-5_2

electrometer in 1876 to capture animal heart ECG waveforms. Notably, in 1887, Waller harnessed a capillary electrometer with dual electrodes—one on the anterior chest and another on the back—to capture human heart contractions' synchronized electrical patterns, thereby crafting the human ECG.

Einthoven, guided by his predecessors' pioneering work, refined the capillary electrometer in 1895, leading to the identification of five distinct cardiac waves, christened as P, Q, R, S, and T waves. This nomenclature system remains in contemporary ECG practice. In 1901, Einthoven elevated the ECG's practical utility by enhancing the string galvanometer (Fig. 2.1), a development that propelled the ECG into a potent tool for cardiovascular disease management. This innovation marked the beginning of ECG's clinical application, embarking on a journey to reshape the landscape of cardiovascular diagnosis and treatment.

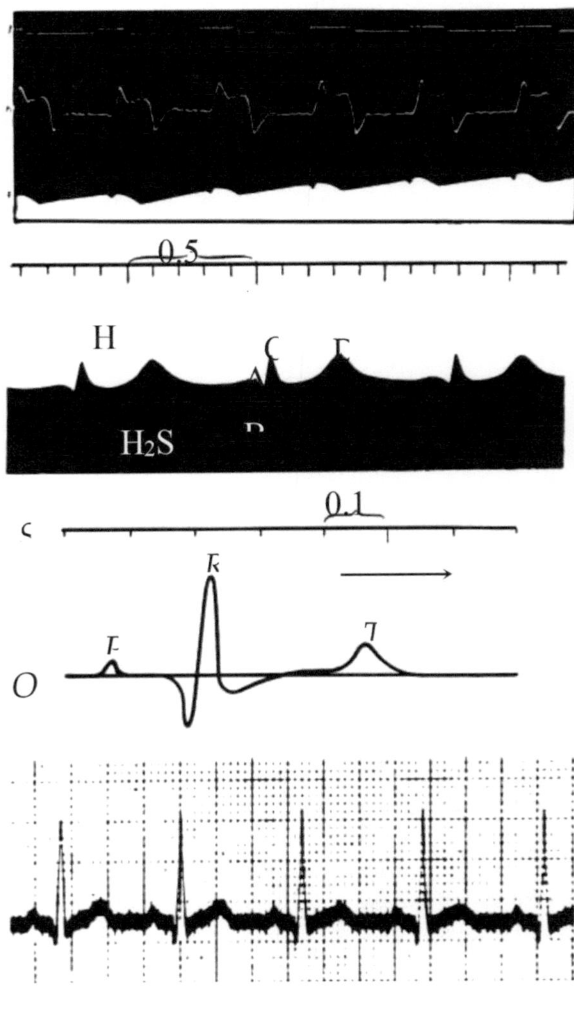


**Fig. 2.1** It illustrates the evolutionary progression of ECG signal acquisition: the top segment displays the ECG signals collected by Waller, the middle segment showcases ECG signals gathered by Einthoven utilizing an upgraded capillary electrometer, while the lower segment portrays ECG signals collected by a string galvanometer

## 2.2 Evolution and Advancements in ECG Equipment and Theory

Kang-Yin Chen and Hua-Yue Tao

### 2.2.1 String ECG Machine

The use of string ECG machine marked a leap in ECG recording technology. Prior to this innovation, Waller's capillary electrometer had been employed for ECG signal recording. However, the capillary electrometer suffered from limitations due to the inertia and friction of capillary mercury columns, resulting in unstable patterns unsuitable for clinical use. Inspired by the string galvanometer, Einthoven wanted to further enhance the string electrocardiograph. Despite its substantial bulk—weighing 270 kg and spanning two rooms—the string ECG machine's standout feature was the incorporation of a 500-fold magnification microscope. This innovation enabled the clear and stable capture of faint cardiac electrical signals. In 1903, Einthoven's publication titled *A New Type of Galvanometer* marked the formal establishment of the string ECG machine as a practical recording device, heralding the official commencement of ECG's clinical application. This breakthrough reached China when Peking Union Medical College Hospital procured two string ECG machines in 1928, inaugurating the utilization of ECG technology within the country.

The application of the ECG machine spurred the progressive refinement of electrocardiography theory. In 1908, Einthoven introduced the concept of standard limb leads, whereby the sequential connection of the patient's left arm, right arm, and left lower limb electrodes could form a heart point equilateral triangle. This electrode configuration facilitated the recording of I, II, and III standard limb lead ECG signals. The adoption of bipolar standard limb lead ECG became standard practice in clinical settings for over two decades. In 1920, Lewis proposed a modification to the bipolar standard limb lead system. Lewis recognized that limb leads were distant from the heart, yielding weak signals that primarily reflected the cardioelectric vector's change in the coronary position; thereby, he designed a unipolar probe electrode, which was placed on the anterior chest, supplemented by the three limb leads, with the dry electrode serving as the central electrical terminal.

Further advancements emerged in 1933 when Wilson refined Lewis's theory, leading to the establishment of the 12-lead ECG system. However, Wilson's 12-lead ECG system exhibited notable deficiencies, such as low voltage in leads aVR, aVL, and aVF, which hindered observation and measurement. A breakthrough emerged in 1942 with Goldberger's proposal. Goldberger suggested disconnecting the limb when recording unipolar limb lead (aVR, aVL, aVF) ECGs, forming a dry electrode connection with the other two limb leads. This approach substantially elevated the voltage of unipolar pressurized limb leads aVL, aVR, and aVF. As a result, unipolar pressurized limb leads aVL, aVR, and aVF were established, a configuration that remains in use to this day.

### 2.2.2 Transition to Electron Tube and Transistor ECG Machines

Following Einthoven's string ECG machine, the evolution of ECG technology continued to unfold. Before the 1950s, significant strides were made in the field of ECG machines due to the advent of electron tubes and transistors. In 1921, German companies Siemens and Holks took the lead in integrating vacuum tube and oscilloscope technologies, resulting in heightened sensitivity, reduced machine size, and the introduction of signal recording displays. These advancements allowed the device to be mounted on a four-wheeled medical cart. By 1930, a design that allowed the instrument to be packed within a portable operating box, enabling doctors to carry it to patients' homes for use. Siemens further pushed the boundaries by producing the first electron-tube enlarged ECG machine in 1934, albeit at a price equivalent to that of a luxury villa. Remarkably, by 1938, the smallest ECG machine weighed a mere 14 kg.

Concurrently, the methodology for recording ECGs had undergone a dramatic transformation. Early ECGs relied on expensive and time-consuming photographic technology. However, in 1932, Swiss scientist Duchosal devised a recording pen, marking a significant step forward. Post-1945, with the application of servo electronics technology, issues of distortion were effectively resolved, and pen recording gained widespread adoption due to its cost-effectiveness and real-time capabilities. Consequently, ECG examinations became characterized by real-time, convenience, and affordability.

The post-1945 era witnessed further advancements. As amplifier circuits matured and differential amplifiers emerged, the ECG machine's anti-interference capabilities saw substantial enhancement. The march of progress ushered in the era of transistors gradually supplanting tubes and integrated circuits succeeding transistors. ECG machines continued to evolve, becoming smaller, lighter, and adaptable to various power supplies, including AC, DC, and battery power, freeing portable ECG inspections from specific conditions.

After the establishment of the People's Republic of China, significant strides were also made in domestic ECG machine research and development. Notably, in 1958, the Shanghai Medical Electronic Instrument Factory successfully produced 409 vacuum tube ECG machines, ending China's reliance on imported ECG machines. Subsequent breakthroughs included the development of the type 7121 ECG machine in 1961, which featured improvements in heat pens and transmission structures, thereby enhancing performance and stability. The 1969 achievement of a transistor and tube hybrid ECG machine marked further advancements in performance, quality, and the machine's weight and size. In the 1970s, domestic research and development of integrated circuit-based ECG machines made remarkable strides, contributing to China's efforts to catch up with the advanced pace set by international counterparts. These accomplishments have played a vital role in improving people's health and well-being during challenging times.

### 2.2.3 Emergence of Digital ECG Machines

The conventional analog signal ECG machines relied on analog amplification signals, employing analog filters to mitigate alternating current interference. However, the cutoff frequency of traditional ECG machines was typically set around 40 Hz, resulting in distortion in the recorded ECG signals, particularly affecting high-frequency components. Furthermore, the long-term preservation of ECG data, crucial for clinical and scientific research, posed challenges due to fading thermal paper printing and the need for manual measurement and analysis.

Following the 1970s and the growing influence of computer applications, digital ECG machines emerged as a significant innovation. Distinct from their analog counterparts, digital ECG machines were equipped with analog-to-digital converters, microprocessors, and digital recording mechanisms. This enabled the collection of ECG signals for digital conversion, analysis, processing, and tracing output. Subsequent advancements incorporated features like liquid crystal displays, various communication ports, and automatic detection of ECG parameters.

Digital ECG machines retained the advantages of analog signal ECG machines, ensuring accurate and complete recording of ECG waveforms. Notably, enhancements were made to improve equipment reproducibility and flexibility, such as eliminating R-wave distortion caused by damping and mitigating electromagnetic interference to achieve uniform waveform display. Other improvements included addressing low-frequency response recording issues, extending the equipment's frequency response range by 150 Hz, and enhancing digital filtering for precise removal of respiration and myoelectric effects, resulting in clearer and more accurate ECG waveforms.

Crucially, digital ECG machines allowed for instant playback, permanent preservation, real-time transmission, and distortion-free signal collection. Beginning in the 1980s, with the integration of large-scale circuits and computer chips, along with advancements in software research and development, the synchronous 12-lead ECG became a powerful tool for diagnosing complex arrhythmias in clinical settings. Additionally, the invention of digital ECG machines facilitated the development and application of 24-h dynamic ECG, various ECG monitoring equipment, ECG mapping systems, signal-averaged ECGs, and other ECG derivative technologies, thus expanding the horizons of electrocardiology's clinical applications.

### 2.2.4 Evolution of ECG Automatic Diagnostic Procedures and Systems

The development of automatic diagnostic programs for ECG is a crucial component of digital ECG machines. With the increasing application of ECG in clinical settings, the need for ECG interpretation by numerous cardiologists or ECG specialists has become a challenge. ECG automatic diagnostic programs offer a successful example in the realm of computer medicine, enhancing efficiency for doctors in performing mundane pattern recognition tasks. This is particularly significant in the analysis of long-term ECG results, such as Holter monitoring. These programs boast high reading speed and precision, with accuracy surpassing manual measurement by tenfold in milliseconds. They also ensure uniform interpretation standards, effectively mitigating human interference.

The inception of ECG automatic diagnostic procedures can be traced back to the late 1950s, when scientists began developing methods for processing ECG data. In 1959, Pipberger presented an electrical automatic diagnostic model for heart data processing. The first dedicated ECG waveform automatic recognition system was established in 1960, marking the official commencement of ECG automatic diagnosis and analysis system development. By the 1970s, commercial ECG automatic diagnosis centers appeared in Europe and the United States. These centers utilized advanced computer equipment and ECG automatic analysis software, enabling remote automatic diagnosis via telephone lines. Such centers could diagnose over 1.4 million ECGs annually. The International Society for Computerized Electrocardiology (ISCE), founded in 1984, holds annual conferences on computer ECG applications to showcase the latest research outcomes in the field.

The ECG automated analysis process comprises three main stages:

1. ECG signal preprocessing, involving filtering processing to mitigate various interference signals like power frequency, myoelectric, and power supply interferences.
2. Waveform detection, identifying and calculating characteristic ECG parameters such as heart rate, PR interval, QRS duration, ST segment, and QT interval.
3. ECG diagnosis, referencing the automatic ECG measurements and judgment criteria to provide corresponding diagnoses based on medical knowledge.

Accurate waveform detection is paramount for obtaining correct diagnoses. Currently, the majority of ECG machines utilize the diagnostic standards recommended by the American College of Cardiology (AHA).

In the 1970s, commercial ECG automatic diagnosis software emerged, with companies like HP, Marquette, Telemed, and Toshiba being pioneers in the field. Over the decades, the main foreign ECG analysis programs include Philips' DXL ECG algorithm, GE's Marquette 12SL ECG analysis software, Glasgow 12-lead ECG analysis software, Japan Fotona's advanced ECG analysis system (Ver.S2), and Nihon Kohden's electrocardiogram analysis system (ECAPS) 12C. In China, the main programs include Libang's Intelligent ECG measurement and analysis program, Coman's ECG 8.0 automatic analysis software, Mindray's Glasgow algorithm, and more. While China's ECG automatic diagnostic program development started later and commercial procedures are comparatively lagging, recent years have seen some companies, such as Libang and Coman, focus on the development and continuous iteration of ECG diagnostic programs with independent intellectual property rights. They have made significant progress in software performance and reliability.

## 2.3 Future Directions of ECG Equipment Development

Kang-Yin Chen and Hua-Yue Tao

### 2.3.1 Wearable ECG Equipment

Wearable ECG devices refer to devices that can be worn directly on the human body to achieve continuous and long-term monitoring of ECG signals. This technology has emerged as a consequence of the digital transformation and miniaturization of ECG equipment. With the current high prevalence of cardiovascular diseases, an aging population, and the relative shortage of medical resources, wearable ECG equipment addresses a substantial societal need and holds promising applications. The development of wearable ECG devices can effectively conserve medical resources and facilitate the shift from a disease diagnosis and treatment-oriented approach to a preventive health-based approach.

The inception of wearable ECG technology can be traced back to dynamic ECG monitoring. In 1961, American biophysicist Holter invented a portable ECG monitoring device that weighed around 1 kg. This device recorded ECG information over several hours using tape, enabling out-of-hospital dynamic ECG monitoring. This breakthrough marked great advancement in the field of ECG monitoring.

The 1990s saw increasing interest in wearable ECG equipment due to advancements in materials, electronics, information technology, and AI. The first interactive wearable system, Smart Shirt, was developed in 1999 by Gopalsamy and others. In the twenty-first century, and especially in recent years, wearable ECG devices have proliferated. Contemporary wearable devices consist of four main components: the signal perception layer, data transmission layer, signal processing layer, and information feedback layer.

- Signal Perception Layer: This layer collects ECG information using electrodes attached to the skin.
- Data Transmission Layer: Responsible for wirelessly transmitting ECG data to mobile devices or cloud servers using technologies like Wi-Fi and Bluetooth.
- Signal Processing Layer: Filters, extracts features, organizes, and classifies ECG signals. It employs methods such as big data and AI for analysis and diagnosis.
- Information Feedback Layer: Communicates the ECG signal diagnosis results to medical institutions and patients, facilitating doctor-patient interaction.

These wearable ECG devices provide an efficient and convenient means of monitoring cardiovascular health, enabling early detection of anomalies and timely medical intervention.

In 2014, the U.S. Food and Drug Administration (FDA) granted approval to AliveCor's Kardia Mobile, marking the entry of wearable ECG devices into the era of medical-grade products. Kardia Mobile utilizes a mobile phone and allows users to touch electrodes on both sides of their fingers to collect ECG information for up to 30 s. It can detect three types of arrhythmias: atrial fibrillation, bradycardia, and tachycardia.

With the increasing popularity of wearable devices like the Apple Watch, AliveCor developed the KardiaBand, which is compatible with the Apple Watch. FDA approval for the Kardia Band was obtained in 2017. This band adds an electrode sensor to the Apple Watch band, enabling users to place an unworn finger on the electrode for data collection. The collected data is then sent to the Apple Watch via Bluetooth connection, where the ECG is displayed on the screen.

The accuracy of monitoring results in wearable ECG devices is closely related to the number of monitoring leads. However, increasing the number of leads, especially those on the chest, may conflict with device miniaturization and patient comfort. Single-lead, three-lead, and twelve-lead wearable ECG devices have been developed and marketed.

Single-Lead Devices: These are typically small and often in a patch design. They simulate a chest triple lead or a limb single lead. While they provide limited information compared to multi-lead devices, they are comfortable and convenient. Examples include AliveCor's Kardia Mobile and KardiaBand.

- Three-Lead Devices: These simulate the chest or limb triple lead and offer more ECG information. They are effective in diagnosing most arrhythmias. BORSA M's iTengo Patch Plus and Heal Force's Prince 180B are examples of these devices.
- Twelve-Lead Devices: Detection of complex conditions like myocardial ischemia often requires a twelve-lead ECG. Although these devices are still more intricate, they offer improved comfort due to the use of dry electrodes. Examples include Master Caution's ECG T-shirt and SmartVest developed by Lenovo.

Current wearable ECG devices estimate heart rate using blood volume map sensors, and accuracy relies on proper skin contact. However, daily usage introduces various interferences such as sound, electricity, and movement, affecting signal collection and interpretation. In future research and development, striking a balance between wearability, signal stability, and reliability remains an urgent challenge (Figs. 2.2 and 2.3).

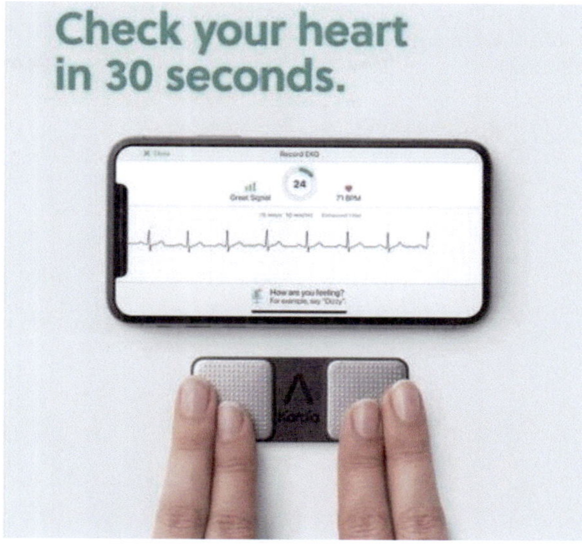


**Fig. 2.2** AliveCor's Kardia Mobile (image from AliveCor)

### 2.3.2 AI-ECG Integration

The convergence of AI and ECG technology stands out as a significant trajectory within the medical domain. Recent years have witnessed the escalating prominence of ECG as a focal point of research, leading to a cascade of compelling findings. Although the inception of AI traces back to the late 1950s, its practical implementation was hampered by model uncertainties, delaying its effective deployment. Following periods of slower advancement in the 1970s and early 1990s, AI underwent a transformative breakthrough in 1997 with IBM's Deep Blue defeating the world chess champion, capturing global attention and marking a milestone in AI's evolution. Within the medical realm, AI's progression has encompassed three distinct phases: the utilization of expert systems for diagnostic approaches, the incorporation of fuzzy logic into diagnostic methodologies, and the adoption of neural networks as a cornerstone of diagnostic methods.

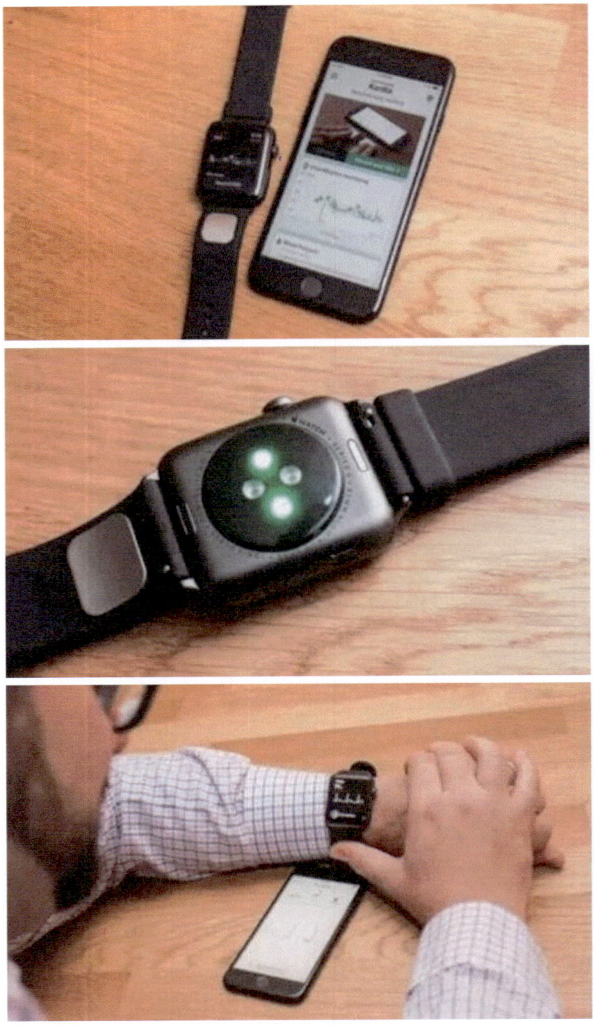

**Fig. 2.3** AliveCor's Kardia Band (image from AliveCor)

# Clinical Application of AI-ECG

# 3

Zheng-Kai Xue, Kang-Yin Chen, Xin-Mu Li, Tong Liu, Jia-Wei Xie, Shao-Hua Guo, Wen-Hua Song, Hui-Min Chu, Guo-Hua Fu, Ni-Xiao Zhang, Bin Zhou, Min Tang, Bin-Hao Wang, Bing-Xin Xie, Guan-Yu Mu, and Peng Wang

## 3.1 Introduction

Xue Zhengkai and Kangyin Chen

The integration of AI into ECG signifies a pivotal shift in the cardiovascular domain. Recent years have borne witness to the advancements of ECG interpretation using AI techniques as a pivotal focus of research, including deep learning and CNN. Multi-layer AI networks excel in detecting intricate signals and patterns that often mimic human perception. A plethora of digitized clinical ECG datasets have provided the foundation for developing AI models, enabling the detection of paroxysmal atrial fibrillation, left ventricular dysfunction, cardiomyopathy, and phenotypes such as hyperkalemia and valve irregularities. This chapter encapsulates the present state of AI-ECG application in cardiovascular disease detection, deliberates its clinical significance, appraises potential limitations, and contemplates future prospects.

ECG, a widely embraced diagnostic method in clinical practice, boasts attributes of non-invasiveness, rapidity, convenience, and cost-effectiveness. In modern medi-

Z.-K. Xue (✉) · K.-Y. Chen · X.-M. Li · J.-W. Xie · S.-H. Guo · W.-H. Song · N.-X. Zhang · B.-X. Xie · G.-Y. Mu · P. Wang
The Second Hospital of Tianjin Medical University, Tianjin, China
e-mail: xvezk2022@tmu.edu.cn; guoshaohua@tmu.edu.cn; songwenhua@tmu.edu.cn; wangpeng123@tmu.edu.cn

T. Liu
Department of Cardiology, Second Hospital of Tianjin Medical University, President of Tianjin Institute of Cardiology, Tianjin, China

H.-M. Chu · G.-H. Fu · B.-H. Wang
The First Affiliated Hospital of Ningbo University, Zhejiang, China

B. Zhou · M. Tang
Fuwai Hospital Chinese Academy of Medical Sciences, Beijing, China

© The Author(s), under exclusive license to Springer Nature Singapore Pte Ltd. 2024

K.-Y. Chen et al. (eds.), *AI Augmented ECG Technology*,
https://doi.org/10.1007/978-981-97-8359-5_3

cine, the 12-lead ECG has emerged as a cornerstone diagnostic tool, providing insights into the heart's physiological, systemic conditions, and structural morphology. With the worldwide prevalence of ECG usage, swift and precise ECG interpretation holds profound implications for disease diagnosis and treatment.

While the ECG procedure has been standardized, the interpretation thereof by medical professionals varies widely based on expertise and experience. Computer-aided ECG diagnosis first emerged in the 1970s, enhancing ECG measurement, analysis, and swift report generation. Across five decades, computer-aided interpretation has evolved into an integral facet of cardiovascular clinical workflow, serving as a pivotal adjunct for ECG analysis. However, computer-generated interpretations, reliant on predefined rules and manually recognized feature patterns, occasionally fail to capture the complexities of ECG signals, leading to notable misdiagnosis rates.

The confluence of digital medicine and AI raises further discussion regarding intelligent healthcare. Recent years have witnessed a surging exploration of AI applications, spanning supervised machine learning to unsupervised deep learning, across various cardiovascular domains [1]. AI, epitomized by deep learning CNNs, has been permeating various aspects of clinical cardiology, including ECG analysis [2]. In comparison to traditional rule-based interpretations, AI-augmented ECG analysis yields superior diagnostic accuracy and operational efficiency [3].

In actuality, raw ECG data, preserved and transmitted in a digital format, constitutes an ideal dataset for AI learning [1]. Extensive repositories utilizing ECG and clinical datasets, alongside studies leveraging substantial computational resources, have vividly showcased the robust efficacy of AI. The software algorithms crafted through AI, when integrated with ECG, significantly amplify the processing capabilities for vast volumes of ECG data. This combination unveils patterns that may not be noticeable to the human eye and enables the precise diagnosis of specific diseases, with a markedly superior accuracy compared to that of clinicians [4]. The surge in computational power and the concurrent expansion of data availability are fundamentally reshaping the role of ECG within modern medicine, ushering further development in ECG technology. In recent years, noteworthy AI applications within the domain of ECG have been documented in a range of cardiovascular journals such as *Nature Medicine*, *The Lancet*, *European Heart Journal*, and *Circulation*. The confluence of augmented computing power and data availability is orchestrating a shift in ECG's role within modern medicine, marking the advent of a new ECG era. Within this chapter, our focus centers on the clinical integration of AI within cardiovascular disease, elucidating the numerous challenges and future prospects for ECG development.

### 3.1.1 AI-ECG

The use of utilization of AI algorithms in the realm of ECG analysis technology aims to improve disease identification, population classification, and thereby aiding clinical decision-making.

In recent years, AI has emerged as a prominent term, often dubbed the "fourth industrial revolution" in the era of extensive data [5]. AI constitutes a computer program that simulates human-like intelligent behavior, meaning the capacity of machines to execute tasks specified by human, such as problem-solving and pattern recognition. As such a program is exposed to vast data repositories and prompted to independently discern patterns, the algorithm begins to discern associations between specific attributes and fundamental facts, even amidst increasingly intricate and nonlinear relationships. This phenomenon is the foundation of machine learning.

Machine learning embodies the aptitude of computers to enhance their knowledge without explicit programming. It encompasses a class of algorithms endeavoring to extract concealed patterns from substantial historical data, subsequently employing these patterns for predictions or categorizations. To elaborate, machine learning can be conceptualized as discovering a function that processes input data and produces the desired outcome, albeit a function too intricate for easy formalization.

Neural networks (NNs) constitute machine learning techniques mirroring the architecture of neurons and NNs in the human brain. Deep learning, a subset of machine learning, employs multi-layer NNs (hence the term "deep") to acquire insights into functions linking input and output sets. Training is achieved by presenting the network with input data alongside corresponding output labels. The model learns distinct rules by adjusting network weights to minimize the error function until the model's output closely approximates actual data values. The potency of deep NNs is rooted in their ability to uncover novel relationships within data, independent of features selected by humans.

Conventional computer models execute ECG analysis with inputs based on morphological and temporal attributes such as QT, QRS, and RR intervals, or QRS and T-wave morphology, yielding outputs like ECG rhythm, blood potassium levels, or left ventricular ejection fraction (EF). Given that the input relies on human-selected features, the model's capability is restricted to those features. In contrast, within a deep learning network, input attributes are autonomously learned by the deep network itself. Employing deep learning, models acquire representations of input data that encompass clinical details concerning the disease, eliminating human biases and the necessity for human feature selection and design, which can be time-consuming, imprecise, and reliant on expertise and knowledge.

### 3.1.2 AI-ECG Application

The initial pursuit in integrating AI with ECG interpretation involves the creation of comprehensive AI models that mimic human interpretive capabilities. Numerous research groups are already engaged in crafting AI-powered algorithms, some of which are undergoing preliminary clinical trials. Given the vast quantities of literature in the field of AI-ECG, this chapter seeks to provide an overview of the current status of AI-ECG development, considering both publication timelines and disease classification.

#### 3.1.2.1 AI-ECG Screening for Cardiac Systolic and Diastolic Dysfunction

In 2018, *Journal of the American College of Cardiology* (*JACC*) published "Application of Machine Learning in ECG Diagnosis of Early Left Ventricular Diastolic Dysfunction" [6]. Sengupta et al. [7] tackled the diagnosis of left ventricular diastolic dysfunction (LVDD) in the context of coronary artery stenosis. Utilizing advanced signal processing and machine learning techniques, the researchers deconstructed ECG signals through a Fourier-like analysis and represented them graphically as signal frequency over time. Applying a machine learning algorithm to these processed ECG features, the model detected LVDD with impressive accuracy, specifically identifying 82% of patients with significant coronary artery stenosis. The study demonstrated good sensitivity (80%) and specificity (84%) in diagnosing LVDD, showing better performance in elderly, hypertensive, and obese patients.

This study exemplifies the early integration of machine learning into ECG analysis, revealing the potential to extract rich information from ECGs beyond visual interpretations, thereby expanding the diagnostic capacity of the conventional 12-lead ECG. Machine learning transcends basic data processing, venturing into the realm of AI, where computers employ logic for inferential operations, identifying important data points from a multitude of ECG-derived features. Although the scope of this research is limited, machine learning holds potential, particularly in handling large, intricate datasets.

In 2019, Attia et al. [8] published a letter in *Nature Medicine*, employing a large CNN model trained on paired 12-lead ECG and echocardiographic data from 44,959 patients. This AI model effectively identified systolic dysfunction using only ECG data. Tested on 52,870 patients, the AI model demonstrated exceptional performance, achieving an AUC of 0.93 along with sensitivity, specificity, and accuracy rates of 86.3%, 85.7%, and 85.7%, respectively. Notably, patients who were screened positive for AI but were confirmed free of ventricular dysfunction exhibited a fourfold higher risk of future dysfunction (hazard ratio (HR): 4.1, 95% confidence interval (CI): 3.3–5.0).

This study showcased the potential of AI in larger-scale ECG analysis, positioning the ECG as a potent screening tool for asymptomatic left ventricular dysfunction (ALVD), even predicting individuals at risk of progressing to low EF with ventricular systolic dysfunction. The AI model detected subtle subclinical, metabolic, or structural abnormalities manifested early in the ECG. However, the applicability of screenings or drug treatments for preventing ventricular dysfunction remains uncertain.

In 2020, the JACC published a machine learning model crafted by Kagiyama et al. [9]. This model utilized both clinical and ECG variables to quantitatively evaluate myocardial diastolic function, specifically targeting the identification of left ventricular diastolic dysfunction. The research endeavor encompassed a multicenter prospective study across four institutions in North America, enlisting a total of 1202 participants. From these participants, 814 individuals hailing from three institutions constituted an internal cohort, randomly divided into a training group and an internal testing group (in an 80:20 ratio). Data from the fourth institution were retained as an external testset ($n = 388$) to gauge the model's generalizability.

The machine learning model underwent development using signal processing ECG, conventional ECG data, and clinical variables. Subsequently, it was rigorously evaluated using the designated test set. The model demonstrated its capacity to predict quantitative values of left ventricular diastolic velocity ($e'$), a metric derived from echocardiography. Notably, the machine learning model exhibited noteworthy performance in both the internal and external test sets, with mean absolute errors of 1.46 cm/s and 1.93 cm/s, respectively. Moreover, the adjusted R-squared values were 0.57 and 0.46, respectively, indicating the model's adeptness in capturing variability in diastolic function.

By synergizing clinical and ECG variables, this study engineered a robust machine learning model capable of furnishing quantitative forecasts regarding myocardial diastolic function. The model's reliance on readily accessible clinical and ECG features represents a cost-effective approach. This strategy could potentially serve as an initial step in the evaluation of left ventricular dysfunction, ultimately contributing to the early diagnosis and improved treatment of patients afflicted with heart failure.

#### 3.1.2.2 AI-ECG Diagnosis of Arrhythmias

A significant upsurge in AI-ECG research was prompted by a 2019 *Lancet* publication, authored by Attia [10–12], which ignited a surge of interest. Attia et al. collected standard 10-s 12-lead ECG data and developed an AI network utilizing CNN to detect ECG characteristics indicative of atrial fibrillation within normal sinus rhythm. Their approach involved categorizing patients with at least one ECG showing atrial fibrillation or atrial flutter as positive for atrial fibrillation. A comprehensive analysis involved 649,931 ECGs of normal sinus rhythm from 180,922 patients, distributed across training, internal validation, and testing datasets in ratios of 7:1:2. The rhythm labels were meticulously assigned under cardiologist supervision. Among the tested patients, 3051 (8.4%) were confirmed to have atrial fibrillation prior to model assessment.

The AI-ECG model demonstrated promising diagnostic performance, yielding an AUC of 0.87 (95% CI: 0.86–0.88), sensitivity of 79.0%, specificity of 79.5%, F1 score of 39.2%, and overall accuracy of 79.4% for single-lead diagnosis of atrial fibrillation. Incorporating ECGs from 31 days preceding the study or the initial recorded atrial fibrillation ECG improved AUC to 0.90, sensitivity to 82.3%, specificity to 83.4%, F1 score to 45.4%, and overall accuracy to 83.3%. Utilizing a substantial number of ECGs as a sample for machine learning and normative external validation, the study showcased AI's ability to detect atrial fibrillation within sinus rhythm. The authors postulated that AI models trained to discern atrial fibrillation's features resulting from changes in atrial structure could establish a foundation for further AI-ECG advancements.

In the same year, Hannu et al.presented a type of DNN that they developed in an article of *Nature Medicine* [13]. They employed 91,232 single-lead ECGs from 53,549 patients who wore ambulatory ECG monitors, aiming to classify 12 rhythm categories. This DNN exhibited remarkable diagnostic prowess, achieving an average F1 score of 0.837, surpassing that of general cardiologists (0.780). In another study published in *Nature Communications* in 2020, Ribeiro et al. [14] introduced a DNN model trained on a dataset encompassing over 2 million labels. This DNN outperformed cardiology residents in recognizing six abnormalities in 12-lead ECG records, yielding F1 scores exceeding 80% and specificity over 99%. This study highlighted the potential of DNN-based ECG analysis to effectively generalize from single-lead to 12-lead examinations, edging closer to integration into standard clinical practices.

#### 3.1.2.3 AI-ECG Predicts Acute Coronary Syndrome

In a 2020 *Nature Communications* article, Al-Zaiti et al. [15] conducted a study utilizing a machine learning-based approach to predict potential acute myocardial ischemia in patients presenting with chest pain. Their approach involved training and testing multiple classifiers using 554 temporal and spatial features extracted from 12-lead ECGs. The study encompassed independent prospective patient cohorts totaling 1244 individuals. The final AI fusion model achieved a substantial 52% improvement in sensitivity compared to commercial interpretation software and a 37% improvement compared to experienced clinicians. Even after excluding cases of ST-elevation myocardial infarction (MI), the model continued to outperform experienced clinicians and commercial ECG software in predicting non-ST-elevation acute coronary syndrome events. This comprehensive study confirmed the value of temporal and spatial ECG features for training AI models and provided a better understanding of rapid and accurate acute coronary syndrome diagnosis.

#### 3.1.2.4 AI-ECG Detection of Cardiomyopathy

A study published in JACC in 2020 by Ko et al. [16] presented a 12-lead ECG-based AI method for detecting hypertrophic cardiomyopathy (HCM). The research involved 2448 patients diagnosed with HCM and 51,153 age- and gender-matched controls. They trained and validated the CNN using digital 12-lead ECGs and then tested the CNN on separate datasets containing 612 patients with HCM and 12,788 control subjects. The CNN demonstrated promising diagnostic capability, achieving an AUC of 0.96, sensitivity of 87%, and specificity of 90% for detecting HCM.

HCM is a relatively rare but significant cause of sudden cardiac death. In many cases, the diagnosis of HCM is confirmed through the use of echocardiography in combination with a patient's clinical history. However, performing echocardiography on a wide scale to detect HCM in asymptomatic individuals is impractical due to logistical and resource limitations.

Another group of researchers [17] employed a large 12-lead ECG dataset to train a machine learning model for detecting HCM and other cardiac structural indicators and diseases. This model also exhibited good performance in detecting HCM, achieving an AUC of 0.91. Notably, it also showed promising performance in detecting pulmonary hypertension (AUC 0.94), cardiac amyloidosis (AUC 0.86), and mitral valve prolapse (AUC 0.77).

In 2021, Goto et al. [18] proposed a method for detecting myocardial amyloidosis using an AI model with either ECG or echocardiography as input. These models were trained and validated across multiple academic medical centers, and the C statistics for detecting myocardial amyloidosis ranged from 0.85 to 0.91, 0.89 to 1.00 (ECG), and 0.89 to 1.00 (echocardiography), respectively. ECG pre-screening enhanced the performance of the echocardiogram models.

The success of these AI-ECG models in diagnosing various cardiomyopathies demonstrates the feasibility of AI-based screening for these conditions and offers potential for extending this approach to other rare or complex heart diseases.

#### 3.1.2.5 AI-ECG Screening for Hyperkalemia

In a 2019 JAMA Cardiology article, Galloway et al. [19] introduced a deep learning model designed for non-invasive screening of hyperkalemia using ECG data. The study evaluated the model's effectiveness in detecting elevated blood potassium levels (≥5.5 mmol/L) in patients with chronic kidney disease (CKD). The model was trained on over 1.5 million ECGs from nearly 45,000 patients who were simultaneously assessed for blood potassium levels. The results indicated that the AI model achieved a sensitivity of 90% and a specificity of 89% in an external validation cohort.

This AI-ECG model offers the potential to detect clinically significant hyperkalemia without requiring blood draws, making it valuable for remote patient care. For instance, it could aid in adjusting medication doses, such as diuretics, for heart failure patients, or optimizing hemodialysis scheduling for CKD patients. This approach could potentially extend to the screening of other electrolyte disorders as well.

#### 3.1.2.6 AI-ECG Screening for Heart Valve Disease

A study by Cohen-Shelly et al. [20], published in the *European Heart Journal* in 2021, utilized CNN to develop an AI-ECG model for identifying patients with moderate-to-severe aortic stenosis (AS). The study involved 258,607 adults who underwent both echocardiography and ECG within 180 days. The AI-ECG model demonstrated an AUC of 0.85 for AS detection, along with sensitivity, specificity, and accuracy rates of 78%, 74%, and 74%, respectively. Notably, patients identified as false positives by the AI-ECG model were found to have a higher risk of developing moderate or severe AS within 15 years compared to true negatives.

This study showcases the potential of AI-ECG in screening for valvular heart diseases, including aortic stenosis and other valve abnormalities such as those involving the mitral, tricuspid, and pulmonary valves.

Additionally, various other applications of AI-ECG have been explored in cardiovascular clinical care. These include assessing patient response to cardiac resynchronization therapy, identifying MI, and detecting long QT syndrome, among others [21–26]. These advances highlight the wide-ranging potential of AI-ECG in enhancing diagnosis and treatment across various cardiovascular conditions.

### 3.1.3 Prospects and Challenges of AI-ECG

The application of AI using NNs has already shown its potential in recognizing subtle patterns in complex digital data across various domains, such as image recognition, autonomous vehicles, pathology analysis, speech recognition, language translation, and medical imaging interpretation [27, 28]. Metabolic and structural disturbances associated with heart diseases can lead to detectable changes in the ECG, which can be effectively identified by well-trained NNs. The accessibility of ECG data for developing AI models in comparison to other clinical data sources is expected to accelerate the integration of AI-ECG into clinical practice, thereby enhancing clinical efficiency. The AI-ECG capabilities demonstrated in previous sections have the potential to influence patient care through screening, diagnosis, prediction, personalized treatment selection, and monitoring.

While preliminary data on the performance of AI-ECG algorithms are promising, the meaningfulness of these technologies lies in their ability to improve clinical practice and patient outcomes. Consequently, numerous AI technologies are currently undergoing testing across various clinical applications. An example is the EAGLE trial [29], which employs an ECG-based AI-supported clinical decision-support tool to diagnose early left ventricular dysfunction. This trial's results demonstrated that the AI model increased the rate of diagnosing low ejection fraction (EF) and led to increased echocardiogram utilization in patients identified as having a high likelihood of low EF [30]. The EAGLE trial is significant as it not only validates the utility of AI models but also explores how information from AI can be effectively interpreted and utilized by clinicians. This understanding of the interaction between humans and AI is crucial for implementing AI tools in clinical practice.

Similarly, the Beagle trial, which employs AI algorithms to identify concurrent or recent atrial fibrillation using 12-lead ECGs obtained during normal sinus rhythm, is also underway to evaluate the potential of AI in screening for atrial fibrillation. Despite promising results, the true impact of AI-ECG on clinical care and patient outcomes requires further establishment through rigorous evidence-based research. The interaction between AI and clinicians, as well as addressing potential barriers and opportunities, remains an important aspect of the integration of AI-ECG into clinical practice.

AI holds significant promise, yet it confronts both inquiries and hurdles. First, while models often stem from high-caliber databases containing meticulously acquired ECGs and phenotypically sound patients, their application to ECGs procured in real-world routine clinical practice might yield subpar outcomes. Moreover, even though these models may excel within a particular demographic, they need meticulous assessment for external validity across diverse populations. Second, the complex nature of NNs, while an optimal representation, also embodies non-linearity, with the underlying associations between input and output data remaining unexplained. Consequently, this imparts a "black box" quality to the model, where the rationale behind network decisions eludes human comprehension, thereby posing a challenge to the clinical integration of deep learning. Numerous machine learning algorithms yield outcomes that struggle to consider features of varying demographics, often manifesting as cryptic "black boxes," resistant to interpretation or modification. Similar biases can confine a machine learning model to a specific population, technology device, or clinical protocol encompassed in the training dataset. Hence, the nature of machine learning models, alongside more conventional approaches such as logistic regression, reinforcement learning, and random forest models, persists as a catalyst that informs both research and clinical practice. Third, several deep learning algorithms are susceptible to adversarial perturbations, leading to consistent misclassification of measured parameters when these algorithms identify anomalies imperceptible to the human eye. Additionally, in the realm of AI literature, a lack of transparency regarding the precise link between training and test sets can obscure the evaluation of published works' quality. Finally, akin to other AI-empowered tools, the development of AI-ECG models necessitates substantial datasets for training, validation, and testing. In some instances, collaborative efforts across multiple centers might be required to create high-precision models. During this iterative process and the external validation of any AI-ECG model, substantial volumes of patient data traverse global research teams, thereby amplifying concerns about safeguarding sensitive patient information against potential cyber threats or breaches.

### 3.1.4 Summary and Outlook

In summary, the rapid growth of AI-ECG technology within cardiovascular medicine is undeniable, with the potential of deep learning and AI applied to the ubiquitous ECG becoming increasingly apparent. While still in its early stages, AI-ECG holds immense promise for applications in ECG diagnosis, cardiovascular risk assessment, clinical decision support, event analysis, and more. The ongoing expansion of clinical research will ultimately determine the value and optimal utilization of these AI tools in the clinical setting, unveiling their multifaceted impact that is currently challenging to predict. As is the case with any medical innovation, AI-ECG must undergo rigorous review, testing, and validation, while clinicians need proper training for its effective use. Once integrated into medical practice, AI-ECG has the potential to revolutionize patient care. With further research and exploration in the future, the adoption of AI-based intelligent clinical approaches is poised to transform the landscape of cardiovascular medicine.

## 3.2 Coronary Heart Disease

Xue Zhengkai and Kang-Yin Chen

### 3.2.1 Understanding Coronary Heart Disease

Coronary heart disease (CHD) is often referred to as coronary artery disease (CAD) or ischemic heart disease (IHD). It encompasses both coronary atherosclerotic heart disease and functional alterations in coronary arteries, such as spasms. The term "coronary heart disease" is commonly used interchangeably with "coronary atherosclerotic heart disease," given that coronary atherosclerosis is responsible for the majority (95–99%) of cases involving myocardial ischemia and reduced oxygen supply. CHD is prevalent and associated with high mortality and disability rates in acute coronary events. It stands as a leading cause of death in developed countries and holds the second-highest position in terms of single-disease mortality in China, as indicated by the *China Cardiovascular Health and Disease Report 2020* [31]. The prevalence and mortality rates of CHD are on the rise in China, impacting a younger demographic and posing a significant public health concern. Timely clinical diagnosis and preventive measures are crucial for managing high-risk groups susceptible to CHD.

The pathogenesis of CHD is rooted in the anatomical and physiological characteristics of the heart and its coronary arteries. The coronary arteries supply blood to the heart and are divided into major branches, including the left and right coronary arteries, which further branch into the left anterior descending and left circumflex branches. These branches continue to divide into smaller vessels, any of which can be affected by atherosclerosis. Under normal conditions, there is a dynamic balance between myocardial oxygen demand, coronary blood flow, and oxygen supply. However, lumen stenosis resulting from coronary artery disease disrupts this equilibrium, leading to myocardial ischemia. Prolonged and severe ischemia can cause irreversible cell damage and myocardial necrosis. Ischemic injury affects the sodium-potassium pump function on cell membranes, causing sodium accumulation and potassium leakage. Consequently, the cell membrane's polarization is compromised during rest, and it struggles to depolarize effectively upon excitation, resulting in a phenomenon known as the "injury current." This electrical signal alteration typically manifests as ST-T changes on an ECG, including ST segment depression (horizontal or downward-sloping) and abnormal T wave inversions or flattening. Additionally, myocardial ischemia increases the risk of various arrhythmias.

CHD is commonly categorized based on mechanisms, development rates, and prognoses of myocardial ischemia into chronic stable coronary heart disease (SCAD) and acute coronary syndrome (ACS). SCAD comprises conditions like chronic stable angina pectoris and ischemic cardiomyopathy, as well as the stable course following an ACS event. ACS, on the other hand, is divided based on ECG characteristics during onset into ST elevation myocardial infarction (STEMI), non-ST elevation myocardial infarction (NSTEMI), and unstable angina pectoris (UA). NSTEMI and UA are collectively referred to as non-ST elevation acute coronary syndrome (NSTE-ACS).

### 3.2.2 Benefits of AI-ECG Application

The ECG serves as a rapid, non-invasive, and effective diagnostic tool for assessing a range of heart conditions and gauging cardiovascular risk. The detection of myocardial ischemia, including acute coronary syndrome, MI, and angina pectoris, heavily relies on ECG analysis. By reflecting the heart's electrophysiological state, the ECG contains a wealth of information regarding its functioning. However, interpreting ECG data demands extensive clinical expertise, making it challenging for untrained physicians to harness its full potential. Furthermore, human interpretation of ECGs varies considerably based on experience, leading to issues with reproducibility.

Computer-aided ECG diagnostic systems can provide rapid and accurate analyses of ECG traces, offering diagnostic reports. Nonetheless, these computer-generated interpretations often rely on predefined rules and artificial patterns, which may not capture the intricate complexities present in ECGs, resulting in notable misdiagnosis rates. With the emergence of artificial intelligence, particularly NNs and deep learning techniques, AI has found applications in diverse fields such as computer vision and speech recognition. Similarly, AI has been extended to ECG analysis for patients with coronary heart disease. Recent studies suggest that ECGs hold hidden information beyond even the discernment of trained experts, which, however, can be uncovered by AI. AI networks have the capacity to extract valuable insights from ECG signals in patients with coronary heart disease, enhancing clinical decision-making accuracy and operational efficiency.

### 3.2.3 Progress in AI-ECG Application for CHD Diagnosis

Due to varying terminologies used by different researchers to describe diseases related to CHD, the research from this chapter may overlap or encompass similar disease types. We will focus on three pivotal aspects of coronary heart disease: MI, myocardial ischemia, and relevant research progress.

#### 3.2.3.1 CHD Detection

In 2016, a significant advancement in the automatic diagnosis of CHD was achieved by Davari et al. [32] through an optimized support vector machine (SVM) model. The researchers harnessed diverse features of heart rate variability (HRV) signals from ECG, including time domain, frequency domain, and nonlinear characteristics, to distinguish between normal and coronary heart disease conditions. The algorithm exhibited remarkable performance, accurately detecting CAD from normal ECG with a remarkable accuracy of 99.2%, sensitivity of 98.43%, and specificity of 100%. The utilization of biomedical signal features emerges as a promising approach to predict patients' health status.

In 2017, Altan et al. [33] introduced an innovative application of the deep belief network (DBN) to diagnose coronary heart disease. Their system employed 24-h ECG signals from the PhysioNet database, extracting brief ECG segments lasting 15 s. By employing the Hilbert-Huang transform, the short-term ECG signals were transformed into distinctive features, enabling the differentiation of CAD and non-CAD patients. Remarkably, the DBN-based classification yielded impressive accuracy, specificity, and sensitivity rates of 98.05%, 98.88%, and 96.02%, respectively.

In 2020, Butun et al. [34] applied capsule networks (CapsNet) within NNs for the automated detection of coronary heart disease from ECG signals. Employing

CapsNet, they analyzed ECG segments lasting 2 s (95,300) and 5 s (38,120) from a group of 40 normal subjects and 7 subjects with coronary heart disease. The study achieved exceptional diagnostic accuracy, with 99.44% and 98.62% accuracy rates for the 2-s and 5-s ECG signal groups, respectively. Importantly, the research demonstrated CapsNet's ability to autonomously learn pertinent representations from raw ECG data without requiring manual techniques. This technology could serve as a swift and precise diagnostic tool aiding cardiologists in their clinical practice.

Jahmunah et al. [35] ventured into investigating the potential of the Gabor CNN model for coronary heart disease, MI, and congestive heart failure detection. They leveraged CNN and the unique Gabor CNN model to classify ECG signals across multiple categories, including normal, CAD, MI, and congestive heart failure (CHF). Impressively, both CNN and Gabor CNN models achieved accuracy rates exceeding 98.5% for the four-level classification. The Gabor CNN model showcased superior performance and reduced computational complexity compared to the traditional CNN model. Additionally, Lih et al. [36] contributed to the progress of ECG signal classification. They explored the synergy of CNN and long short-term memory (LSTM) models to categorize ECG signals into CAD, MI, and CHF. Developing a robust 16-layer LSTM model and employing 10-fold cross-validation, their research yielded a classification accuracy of 98%. This achievement underscores the potential of combined models in enhancing diagnostic capabilities for coronary heart disease-related conditions.

#### 3.2.3.2 Detecting MI: Advancements and Breakthroughs

In 2018, researchers from Wuhan University delved into real-time multi-lead CNNs for MI detection [37]. They devised a beat segmentation algorithm to analyze multi-lead ECG signals. These beats underwent fuzzy information granulation (FIG) preprocessing and were then fed into a multi-lead CNN (ML-CNN). Evaluating their approach on a PTB database, they achieved impressive sensitivity (95.40%) and specificity (97.37%), resulting in an accuracy of 96.00%. The study showcased the potential of this technique for mobile medical applications.

In 2020, Al-Zaiti et al. [38] introduced a novel application of 12-lead ECG in predicting acute myocardial ischemia using machine learning. Their models, developed with 554 temporal and spatial features of 12-lead ECGs, underwent rigorous validation through large prospective cohort studies (n = 1244). The model exhibited a remarkable 52% sensitivity improvement over commercial ECG interpretation software and a 37% enhancement over experienced clinicians. Even after excluding ST-segment elevation myocardial infarction (STEMI) cases, the model continued to outperform both software and clinicians in non-ST-segment elevation ACS (NSTE-ACS) events.

Traditional ECG interpretation methods often fall short in detecting MI, whereas AI-powered CNNs excel in recognizing intricate ECG patterns. Makimoto et al. [24] demonstrated this prowess by developing a CNN for identifying MI using the PTB ECG database. This CNN outperformed physicians, significantly enhancing the F1 score and accuracy. Another promising study [23] from Shanghai tenth

People's Hospital showcased an AI-based STEMI diagnostic algorithm that demonstrated superior performance compared to cardiologists.

In 2021, researchers from Taiwan [39] unveiled a deep learning model (DLM) for 12-lead ECG as a diagnostic support tool. The DLM achieved remarkable AUC values, surpassing even the best doctors, and exhibited substantial diagnostic capability for STEMI and non-ST-segment elevation myocardial infarction (NSTEMI) testing, even when combined with conventional cardiac troponin I.

In that same year, another study published in the journal *Frontiers in Cardiovascular Medicine* by researchers from Longhua Central Hospital in Shenzhen [40] presented a NN algorithm for automated diagnosis of acute myocardial infarction (AMI) based on 12-lead ECGs. Leveraging the open-source PTB-XL database for training and validation (sample ratio of 7:3), the study involved 21,837 clinical trials from the PTB-XL dataset. The training and validation subsets included 15,285 training sets and 6552 validation sets, with 205 ECGs randomly selected as test sets from datasets established by Chapman University and Shaoxing People's Hospital. The algorithm achieved impressive AUC values: 0.964 for the training set, 0.944 for the validation set, and 0.977 for the test set. Moreover, it demonstrated high accuracy in localizing different types of AMI, with AUC values ranging from 0.961 to 0.996.

#### 3.2.3.3 Detection of Myocardial Ischemia

A novel approach to the detection of myocardial ischemia was introduced by Hussein et al. [41]. In their method, changes in ischemia-related ECG components, specifically the ST segment and PR segment, were observed using the Choi-Williams time-frequency distribution. Features related to ST and PR intervals were extracted and then fed into a multi-class SVM classifier for training and detecting unknown conditions. This classification process utilized data from 92 healthy individuals and 266 patients from various databases. The model achieved an impressive accuracy of 99.09%, a sensitivity of 99.49%, and a specificity of 98.44%.

Fernandez et al. [42] investigated the classification of non-ischemic heart disease based on Holter ECG records. While Holter records are commonly used to detect transient cardiac events, distinguishing non-ischemic events can be challenging due to false positives stemming from factors like heart rate and electrical axis changes. To address this, researchers enhanced the classification of ischemic and non-ischemic events in long-term ST-segment databases. They introduced new spectral and temporal parameters derived from continuous wavelet transform, including ST-segment level, slope, T-wave width and peak, R-wave peak, and QRS group width. The algorithm's sensitivity and specificity for ischemic and non-ischemic event classification using the nearest neighbor classifier were 84.1% and 92.9%, respectively.

Gumpfer et al. [43] proposed a NN-based algorithm for detecting deep myocardial scar data. The presence of myocardial scarring is indicative of ischemic heart disease development, but its effects on the ECG are often non-specific and difficult for clinicians to discern. The model underwent training and evaluation using 12-lead ECG time series datasets and clinical parameters through sixfold cross-validation.

The model achieved an AUC of 0.89, sensitivity of 70.0%, specificity of 84.3%, and accuracy of 78.0%. The high diagnostic accuracy of this deep learning-based myocardial scar detection model offers a promising and comprehensible approach to myocardial ischemia screening.

Another research team [44] proposed a multi-lead ensemble neural network (MENN) to differentiate between anterior MI and lower MI compared to healthy controls. By combining a three-seed network with multi-lead ECG signals, the researchers harnessed comprehensive ECG information, significantly enhancing classification performance. The sensitivity, specificity, and AUC values for detecting AMI and lower MI were excellent, surpassing 90%, with fivefold cross-validation on the PTB database.

Zeng et al. [45] introduced a novel MI automatic detection technology utilizing hybrid feature extraction and AI tools. Representative features were extracted using wavelet transform, variational mode decomposition, and phase space reconstruction. These features were combined with NNs to model and detect abnormal cardiac system dynamics caused by MI. The model achieved an average classification accuracy of 97.98%, demonstrating its potential as a complementary MI detection algorithm for hospitals, aiding clinicians in confirming diagnoses.

In a study by Cho et al. [25], a deep learning-based AI algorithm (DLA) was developed and validated for detecting MI in 6-lead ECGs. By utilizing a variational autoencoder (VAE), the researchers reconstructed 6-lead ECGs from 6-lead limb ECGs. The AUC values for DLA and VAE were 0.880 and 0.854, respectively, suggesting that MI detection can be extended to 6-lead ECGs.

Addressing the need for improved lead relationships and temporal characteristics in ECG signal analysis, researchers from Chongqing University [46] proposed a multi-lead attention approach (MLA-CNN-BiGRU) that combines CNN and bidirectional gated recurrent units (BiGRU). This approach achieved remarkable accuracy, sensitivity, and specificity, underscoring its potential for accurate MI detection and localization.

Lastly, Sharma et al. [47] developed a diagnostic system for MI using single-channel single-lead ECGs. The system achieved high accuracy rates of 99.62% and 99.74% on noisy and noise-free datasets, respectively, with the implementation of a new two-band optimal biorthogonal filter bank and a K-nearest neighbor algorithm.

These pioneering studies collectively demonstrate the remarkable potential of AI-powered algorithms in enhancing the accuracy, efficiency, and effectiveness of MI diagnosis, ultimately benefiting patient care and clinical decision-making.

### 3.2.4 Prospects and Challenges of AI Application in Coronary Heart Disease

In the realm of CHD, AI algorithms for diagnosis have flourished, encompassing diverse models like waveform conversion, feature extraction, and intelligent filtering. However, the diagnosis of CHD is multifaceted, involving patient symptoms, cardiovascular risk factors, ECG examinations, lab tests, coronary angiography, and more. It necessitates expertise from various disciplines such as anatomy, pathology, and physiology. While effective methods have emerged, AI algorithms often lack prospective testing in real-life medical settings. The reliability and accuracy of these technologies remain uncertain, warranting further validation.

Moreover, many AI algorithms excel in specific ECG types based on limited publicly available datasets. This restricts their generalization capacity, and models built on smaller datasets may suffer from overfitting issues that demand additional validation. Researchers in AI-ECG must straddle medical expertise and cutting-edge technical skills, a demanding combination that presents a challenge.

In summary, AI-ECG holds significant potential and promising prospects in coronary heart disease detection. However, it also inherits the advantages and drawbacks of AI technology itself. As AI continues to evolve through exploration and research, the integration of new AI algorithms with ECG data is poised to bring profound and lasting transformations to CHD diagnosis and the broader cardiovascular domain.

## 3.3 Heart Failure

Xin-Mu Li, Tong Liu, and Jia-Wei Xie

Heart failure (HF) encompasses a range of structural and/or functional abnormalities in the heart. This results in intricate clinical syndromes characterized by ventricular contraction and/or diastolic dysfunction, leading to symptoms such as dyspnea, debilitation, and fluid retention (including pulmonary congestion, systemic congestion, and peripheral edema). Heart failure can be classified based on the left ventricular ejection fraction (LVEF) into heart failure with reduced ejection fraction (HFrEF), preserved ejection fraction (HFpEF), and mid-range ejection fraction (HFmrEF). It is further classified into chronic and acute heart failure based on onset and duration, with acute cases often transitioning into chronic conditions.

Although hospitalization can alleviate symptoms in many acute cases, chronic heart failure can worsen due to various triggers, necessitating recurrent hospitalizations [48]. As a severe manifestation or advanced-stage complication of diverse heart conditions, heart failure carries substantial mortality and readmission rates. The prevalence of heart failure ranges from 1.5% to 2.0% in developed countries, surpassing 10% in individuals aged 70 and older [49]. Globally, over 26 million adults have been diagnosed with heart failure, with 3.6 million new cases added annually [50]. Among them, mortality within a year of diagnosis ranges from 17% to 45%, and the remaining patients succumb within five years. Projections indicate that over 8 million adults will be affected by heart failure by 2030 [51].

Early diagnosis of chronic heart failure holds vital clinical importance due to its irreversible and progressive nature, making it an important focus of discussion and research among clinicians. Currently, common diagnostic methods for cardiovascular diseases encompass ECG, chest X-ray, biomarkers, echocardiography, laboratory tests, etc. ECG, being non-invasive, portable, and user-friendly, plays a crucial role in cardiovascular assessments. Pathophysiological heart changes during heart failure often lead to alterations in its electrical activity, thus making ECG data a potential foundation for early diagnosis and prognosis assessment.

In recent years, AI's rapid advancement has revolutionized the medical field. AI's efficient and convenient data processing empowers clinicians with reliable, evidence-based medical insights, aiding clinical decision-making. This section concentrates on the utilization of AI-driven ECG analysis in heart failure diagnosis and prevention.

## 3.3.1 Diagnosis of Heart Failure

### 3.3.1.1 Heart Rate Variability and Heart Failure Diagnosis

The correlation between heart rate variability (HRV) and heart failure has emerged as a prominent research focus in the field. AI algorithms have been employed to differentiate between healthy individuals and heart failure patients using HRV-related data [52, 53]. Utilizing a publicly available ECG database, researchers have consistently demonstrated favorable model performance. For instance, in 2014, Liu et al. [54] effectively detected congestion in individuals with chronic heart failure (CHF). They combined a support vector machine (SVM) classifier with three non-standard HRV features (SUM_TD, SUM_FD, and SUM_IE) to establish a CHF classification model. The model exhibited remarkable accuracy, sensitivity, and specificity, all reaching 100%. Similarly, a study conducted in 2019 [55] employed long short-term memory (LSTM) network deep learning to identify CHF patients. ECG data from five public databases were utilized for training and testing, categorized based on disease severity, and compared across different RR intervals ($n = 500$, 1000, and 2000). The results demonstrated high accuracy rates of 99.22%, 98.85%, and 98.92% for BIDMC-CHF, NSR, and FD databases, respectively. For NSR-RR and CHF-RR databases, accuracy ranged from 82.51% to 87.55%. While these studies showcase robust model performance, they often prioritize refining machine learning techniques. These algorithms frequently incorporate numerous HRV parameters, enhancing model complexity. However, the relatively modest sample size of the databases employed restricts broader clinical application.

### 3.3.1.2 Traditional Algorithms and Heart Failure Diagnosis

Recent years have witnessed heightened interest in utilizing AI-driven ECG analysis for heart failure detection. In 2016, Masetic and Subasi [56] introduced an automated ECG heartbeat classification system employing machine learning to differentiate normal heartbeats from those indicative of congestive heart failure. ECG data were drawn from the BIDMC Congestive Heart Failure Database and PTB Diagnostic ECG database. The study involved 2800 ECG data samples, with 1500 from congestive heart failure patients and 1300 from normal individuals. Feature extraction employed the autoregressive (AR) Burg method, and classification entailed five distinct classifiers, namely, C4.5 decision tree, k-nearest neighbor (kNN), support vector machine, artificial neural network, and random forest classifier. The random forest classifier exhibited exceptional performance, achieving a classification accuracy of 100% with a corresponding ROC curve and F-value of 1. This study underscores the applicability of machine learning classifiers in the realm of cardiovascular medicine, offering valuable insights for clinical practice.

#### 3.3.1.3 Deep Learning and Heart Failure Diagnosis

Deep learning, a subfield of machine learning, involves neural network structures comprising multiple hidden layers. Despite being in its early stages of development, deep learning has demonstrated significant potential in diagnosing and treating cardiovascular diseases. In 2018, Acharya et al. [57] developed an 11-layer convolutional neural network (CNN) to identify ECG signals from both healthy individuals and CHF patients. Their model's performance was tested across four different datasets, with Group B exhibiting the best results: accuracy, specificity, and sensitivity of 98.97%, 99.01%, and 98.87%, respectively. Although a perfect accuracy of 100% was not achieved, this study marked the pioneering use of CNN models for detecting ECG signals in CHF patients, paving the way for subsequent deep learning advancements. Numerous subsequent studies have further demonstrated the potential of deep learning in heart failure diagnosis.

In 2021, Cho et al. [58] utilized a large dataset of 39,371 12-lead ECGs from 17,127 patients to develop an innovative AI algorithm using CNN. The algorithm's objective was to detect HFrEF where EF < 40%. The study assessed the performance of the algorithm in both internal and external validation cohorts. For HFrEF detection, the AUC of 12-lead ECGs was 0.913 and 0.961 in the respective cohorts, while single-lead ECGs achieved AUC values of 0.874 and 0.929. This study suggests the effectiveness of wearables (which typically utilize a single lead) in screening for HFrEF, potentially preventing disease progression and reducing mortality risk. Additionally, the study highlighted influential factors such as lateral and anterior wall leads and identified correlations with heart rate, QT interval, QRS duration, and T-axis.

The 2016 ESC Guidelines [48] acknowledge the challenge of precisely diagnosing HFpEF, given its normal LVEF and nonspecific symptoms. However, AI-assisted echocardiographic interpretation has made strides in recent years. Chiou et al. [59] developed an AI model for rapid HFpEF screening, achieving accuracy, sensitivity, and specificity of 0.91, 0.96, and 0.85, respectively, with an AUC of up to 0.95. This model screens HFpEF patients using the four-chamber cardiac view in echocardiography, offering a quicker, time-saving, and more accurate approach.

While both traditional machine learning and deep learning algorithms are vital in AI science, deep learning's capacity for feature learning—enabling models to automatically identify necessary features and relationships from raw data—often leads to enhanced performance. For instance, in a study by Kwon et al. [60], a deep learning-based algorithm (DEHF) for heart failure diagnosis surpassed logistic regression (LR) and random forest (RF) algorithms in identifying HFrEF (EF ≤ 40%) and other endpoints. DEHF achieved AUCs of 0.843 and 0.889 in internal and external validation for HFrEF detection, surpassing LR and RF. Another study by Cinar et al. [61] highlighted the classification prowess of deep learning, where LSTM and mixed Alexnet-SVM algorithms achieved accuracy rates of 90.67% and 96.77% in classifying ECG signals of abnormal arrhythmia, congestive heart failure, and normal sinus rhythm, outperforming traditional algorithms.

#### 3.3.1.4 AI-ECG and COVID-19–Related Heart Failure

The COVID-19 pandemic has had a profound impact on global health systems, prompting countries to develop drugs, vaccines, and screening tools. Beyond respiratory symptoms, severe COVID-19 infections can lead to myocarditis, potentially resulting in heart failure and even death. The rapid and accurate diagnosis of such patients is critical.

ELEFT [62], an AI testing software granted emergency use authorization (EUA) by the FDA, specializes in analyzing ECG data to detect patients with a LVEF of 40% or less. This assists clinicians in making informed decisions, including whether an echocardiogram is necessary. However, the software's scope is limited to patients with low LVEF, which often indicates advanced myocardial involvement. Detecting early-stage heart failure necessitates the assessment of left ventricular end-diastolic pressure (LVEDP). Researchers have been dedicated to identifying patients with elevated LVEDP through machine learning algorithms [63], achieving an AUC of up to 0.89. The ongoing enhancement and future application prospects of this technology hold promise for further advancements in early heart failure detection.

The AI-driven analysis of ECG data continues to offer valuable insights in the context of COVID-19, aiding in the prompt identification and management of patients at risk of developing heart failure due to severe infections.

### 3.3.2 Prevention and Treatment of Heart Failure

Deep learning-based ECG analysis models also contribute to the early screening and prevention of heart failure. Asymptomatic left ventricular dysfunction (ALVD) affects 3–6% of the general population, impacting patients' quality of life and potentially raising mortality risks. However, early detection of ALVD offers the chance for effective treatment, emphasizing the need for affordable and non-invasive screening tools.

Attia et al. [8] developed a CNN utilizing data from 12-lead ECGs and echocardiograms of 44,959 patients from the Mayo Clinic to identify individuals with ventricular dysfunction and an ejection fraction (EF) of 35% or less. The model's validation against an independent cohort of 52,870 patients demonstrated an AUC of 0.93, sensitivity of 86.3%, specificity of 85.7%, and accuracy of 85.7%. Among patients without ventricular dysfunction, those who screened positive by AI had a 4.1-fold higher risk of future ventricular dysfunction. To expand the algorithm's application, Jentzer et al. [64] employed the same model to identify patients with left ventricular systolic dysfunction (LVSD, LVEF $\leq$40%) in the cardiac intensive care unit (CICU). The AI-ECG model maintained strong performance, achieving an AUC of 0.83 and an overall accuracy of 76%.

The presence of atrial fibrillation (AF) can affect echocardiographic evaluation of LVEF, influencing treatment decisions for patients. Kashou et al. [65] addressed this issue by applying the model to detect LVSD in AF patients in the CICU. The study encompassed 3780 patients with AF and sinus rhythm who underwent simultaneous ECG and transthoracic echocardiography (TTE). The model's performance exhibited an AUC of 0.79 for LVSD detection in AF patients and 0.82 for those with sinus rhythm. This research showcased the AI-ECG model's potential as a noninvasive, cost-effective, and rapid screening tool for early LVSD detection, particularly in resource-limited settings.

The study by Attia and colleagues, while valuable, had limitations in identifying patients with mild disease or early stages of LV insufficiency, as it focused on screening patients with low EF. To address this gap, Potter et al. [66, 67] redefined left ventricular dysfunction (LVD) using diastolic echocardiographic parameters and global longitudinal strain. This redefinition allowed for early screening and enabled the development of a machine learning random forest (RF) algorithm for LVD detection using a signal-processed "energy waveform" ECG (ewECG). The study involved 398 subjects at risk for heart failure who underwent both ewECG and echocardiography. The RF algorithm demonstrated a sensitivity of 88% and specificity of 70%, outperforming clinical risk scores, biomarkers, and automated ECG analysis algorithms. Remarkably, the use of ewECG in screening individuals at risk of heart failure led to a 45% reduction in the clinical need for echocardiography. If this technology is refined and applied clinically, it has the potential to significantly reduce the medical burden on high-risk individuals and enhance medical resource utilization efficiency.

To further validate the role of AI-ECG in diagnosing and treating patients with clinical heart failure, Yao et al. [29, 68] conducted a randomized clinical trial. The trial aimed to evaluate the efficacy of ECG-based AI screening tools in primary care. ECGs were obtained from 22,641 adults without prior heart failure, with some receiving the AI-based intervention and others serving as controls. The primary outcome was new-onset left ventricular systolic dysfunction with an EF of 50% or less. The AI algorithm was integrated into the electronic health record (EHR) to automatically screen for patients with decreased LVEF and prompt clinicians to obtain transthoracic echocardiography (TTE) for positive cases. The results showed that the diagnosis rate of LVEF decline improved in the intervention group compared to the control group. Among patients with positive AI-ECG results, the diagnosis rate also improved in the intervention group. Additionally, the use of echocardiograms increased in the intervention group for patients with positive AI-ECG results. These findings underscore the potential of AI-based ECG as a powerful screening tool for asymptomatic individuals, facilitating early disease identification. When properly applied to high-risk populations, this technology could lead to enhanced disease prevention, diagnosis, and treatment, with the potential to reduce disease burden and mortality.

Elevated diastolic blood pressure has been identified as a significant contributor to heart failure, even in patients with normal LVEF. Studies have shown that nearly 50% of patients with normal LVEF develop heart failure due to elevated diastolic blood pressure [69]. Additionally, changes in left ventricular diastolic function often precede or coincide with systolic dysfunction in patients with heart failure [70]. Given the importance of LVDD in heart failure management, efforts have been directed toward its early detection and management. Sengupta et al. [7] conducted a groundbreaking study in 2018 using signal-processed ECG (spECG) to predict cardiac diastolic dysfunction. The study achieved an impressive AUC of 0.91, with sensitivity and specificity of 80% and 84%, respectively. Building on this research, a more comprehensive machine learning model was developed in 2020 by the same team [9]. This multicenter prospective study included 1202 participants and aimed to quantitatively predict left ventricular diastolic velocity (*e'*) using spECG, traditional ECG, and clinical data. The model effectively differentiated abnormal myocardial diastole and diastolic dysfunction, showcasing AUC values of 0.83 and 0.76 for the internal test set and 0.84 and 0.80 for the external test set. The model's performance was consistent across different cohorts and regions, suggesting its reliability and potential for clinical application. As an important tool for early diagnosis, this machine learning model has the potential to be enhanced further by incorporating additional echocardiographic parameters, such as left ventricular and left atrial strain. Follow-up data analysis could provide insights into the model's value in assessing prognosis, thereby offering valuable information for heart failure management and treatment decisions. The focus on early detection and management of LVDD demonstrates a significant step toward improving heart failure outcomes.

Cardiac magnetic resonance (CMR) is widely recognized as the gold standard for evaluating ventricular volume, mass, and LVEF, providing crucial information for diagnosing heart failure. However, the high cost and time-consuming nature of CMR limit its widespread use. To address this issue, recent advancements in AI have shown promise in combining ECG data with cardiac structural imaging to improve the detection and diagnosis of cardiovascular conditions. Khurshid et al. [71] introduced a CNN model called "left ventricular mass-AI" (LVM-AI), utilizing ECG data and CMR results from a large cohort of 32,239 UK patients. This model aims to enhance the detection of left ventricular hypertrophy (LVH) by predicting left ventricular (LV) mass based on ECG information. The study demonstrated a strong correlation between LV mass predicted by LVM-AI and LV mass derived from CMR. In the UKBiobank test set, the model achieved substantial predictive power for LVH, reaching an impressive AUC of 3.97 (95% CI: 2.70–5.84). This innovative approach, combining ECG and cardiac structural imaging, holds the potential to revolutionize the diagnosis and prevention of cardiovascular disease, offering a more accessible and cost-effective alternative to traditional CMR.

Furthermore, AI-driven analysis of ECG data offers a novel avenue for tracking blood drug levels among individuals grappling with heart failure. Notably, this application finds significance in the context of digoxin usage. The 2016 ESC guidelines [48] underscore the utility of digoxin in managing ventricular rate for heart failure patients unresponsive to alternative treatments. Additionally, patients experiencing HFrEF and sinus rhythm may find value in digoxin as a means to curtail hospitalization risk, cementing its indispensable role within clinical practice. However, epidemiological investigations highlight that approximately 1% of congestive heart failure (CHF) patients undergoing digoxin therapy experience digoxin intoxication, accentuating a pressing concern [72]. This concern primarily stems from the challenges posed by resource-intensive and time-consuming serological (SDC) testing for assessing digoxin concentrations. This frequently results in instances of either erroneous diagnosis or delayed identification of digoxin poisoning. Yet, the amalgamation of AI algorithms with ECG data introduces a transformative solution to this quandary. To address this issue, DW Chang et al. [73] developed a deep learning model for detecting digoxin poisoning (defined as serum digoxin concentration ≥2 ng/mL) using ECG performance. The study analyzed 61 ECGs from patients with digoxin poisoning and 177,066 ECGs from emergency department patients. The model exhibited impressive diagnostic performance, with an AUC of 0.912 and sensitivity and specificity of 84.6% and 94.6%, respectively. This AI-based approach holds promise for supporting the timely detection of digoxin toxicity in emergency rooms, potentially leading to improved patient outcomes. Moreover, the model's integration into ambulances or remote ECG machines could facilitate telemedicine and extend its reach to underserved areas.

## 3.3.3 Heart Failure Management

### 3.3.3.1 Enhancing Risk Stratification

Heart failure, characterized by its heterogeneous nature, often entails diverse clinical trajectories and prognoses, prompting the imperative for tailored and refined risk stratification strategies in the realm of medical management. While AI models boast exceptional accuracy, their efficacy often hinges on extensive training data, which can be challenging to accumulate promptly within real-world contexts. To address this limitation, Tse et al. [74] devised a multi-task learning paradigm, adept at circumventing data insufficiencies, to effectively forecast adverse outcomes in risk stratification. Incorporating a multitude of factors encompassing baseline variables, laboratory assays, electrocardiographic profiles, and echocardiographic parameters, the study embraced a multimodal approach to evaluate 312 Chinese heart failure patients with an ejection fraction (EF) ≤ 45%. Among them, 76 presented with new-onset atrial fibrillation, 62 endured transient ischemic attacks (TIA) or strokes, and 117 succumbed during follow-up. Age, left atrial storage strain (LARS), and systolic strain (LACS) emerged as pivotal predictors for incident atrial fibrillation, while age and smoking demonstrated prognostic potential for stroke occurrence. Notably, the machine learning model's predictive capacity surpassed that of traditional logistic regression, underscoring its superiority.

Furthermore, Pandey et al. [75] aimed to discern distinct risk tiers within the HFpEF subgroup, employing a deep neural network (DeepNN) model. Successfully discriminating high-risk and low-risk patient clusters with remarkable accuracy, the model's outcomes substantiated the heightened LV filling pressures, augmented admission rates, and elevated mortality rates characterizing the high-risk cohort. Encouragingly, these high-risk individuals displayed enhanced responsiveness to spironolactone treatment relative to their low-risk counterparts. This intricate integration of AI-driven risk stratification holds substantial promise in enriching heart failure management strategies and steering interventions toward those who stand to benefit most.

#### 3.3.3.2 Predicting Prognosis

While significant strides have been made in diagnosing and treating heart failure, patient outcomes remain a challenge, and optimizing management to enhance these outcomes stands as a paramount goal for medical practitioners.

As early as 1995, a seminal study [76] highlighted neural networks' ability to employ echocardiographic data for accurate 1-year mortality predictions in 95 heart failure patients, surpassing linear models and clinical judgments. In more recent times, Bazoukis et al. [77] underscored the pivotal role of machine learning in heart failure diagnosis, management, and prognostication, consistently outperforming traditional techniques. Nevertheless, a JAMA Cardiology publication in 2017 [78] found machine learning algorithms to offer no improvement in forecasting 30-day readmission rates for heart failure compared to conventional predictive models. Bayesian networks, random forest, gradient enhancement, and LASSO model validations yielded C-statistics of 0.618, 0.607, 0.614, 0.624, and 0.618, respectively. To address this, Awan et al. [79] attributed the often unsatisfactory performance of models to class imbalance in medical data, necessitating meticulous model selection and metric choice for heart failure readmission prediction. Awan's team introduced a multi-layer perceptron (MLP)-based model for predicting 30-day readmission or mortality in heart failure patients, demonstrating AUC, sensitivity, and specificity of 0.62, 48%, and 70%, respectively. The model outperformed weighted random forest, weighted decision tree, logistic regression, and weighted support vector machine models. In a recent investigation [80], an analysis of 7516 heart failure patient hospital admissions in New York City over a decade employed an integrated machine learning approach, revealing a differentiation of 0.83 (95% CI: 0.80–0.87) for predicting 30-day post-discharge mortality, compared to a baseline model's 0.79 (95% CI: 0.75–0.84).

Building upon these insights, Jing et al. [81] harnessed a machine learning model with a training dataset from the Geisinger electronic health database. This comprehensive model incorporated 26 clinical variables, 90 diagnostic codes, 41 ECG results, 44 echocardiographic findings, and 8 medical data points, yielding an AUC range of 0.74–0.77. The model forecasted that 2844 of 13,238 patients would experience 1-year mortality, and rectifying the existing care gap could potentially save 231 lives. Notably, this machine learning approach not only stratified at-risk patients but also pinpointed those likely to benefit most from intervention, thus furnishing robust evidence for clinical decision-making enhancements.

#### 3.3.3.3 Heart Failure Management in Complicated Cases

The intricate management of heart failure, a predominant cause of elderly hospitalizations, is influenced by factors such as aging, comorbidities, and frailty. Notably, more than 70% of heart failure patients aged over 80 may exhibit frailty, which some studies suggest can serve as a primary prognostic indicator [48, 82]. Building upon this insight, a pioneering 2021 study [83] devised an electronic frailty index to anticipate short-term mortality in heart failure patients. Key variables like the prognostic nutrition index (PNI), age, and neutrophil-to-lymphocyte ratio (NLR) emerged as vital determinants in forecasting 30- and 90-day heart failure mortality. Leveraging gradient-lifting models, the study achieved commendable predictive performance with AUCs of 0.90 and 0.92 for 30- and 90-day mortality, respectively. Although further validation against comprehensive inflammatory and nutritional indicators is warranted, integrating the straightforward NLR and PNI indices into clinical decision-making is poised to notably enhance efficiency.

The intersection of heart failure and diabetes is widely recognized, bearing a grim prognosis. However, traditional risk prediction models have struggled to precisely gauge heart failure risk in type 2 diabetes patients [84]. To address this technical gap, Segar et al. [85] pioneered a heart failure risk prediction model using a randomized survival forest (RSF) methodology, drawing from data encompassing 8756 participants in the Action to Control Cardiovascular Risk in Diabetes (ACCORD) study. Of these, 319 patients (3.6%) experienced heart failure over a median 4.9-year follow-up. The RSF model not only showcased superior predictive capabilities over Cox regression but also successfully identified heart failure risk predictors. Building on this foundation, the team constructed the WATCH-DM risk score (based on body mass index, age, hypertension, creatinine, HDL-C, diabetes control level, QRS duration, myocardial infarction, and coronary artery bypass grafting event) to project 5-year heart failure risk in type 2 diabetes patients. Categorized into five levels, the risk score revealed an escalating 5-year heart failure risk, ranging from 1.1% in grade 1 (WATCH-DM score $\leq 7$) to 17.4% in grade 5 (WATCH-DM score $\geq 14$) patients.

### 3.3.4 Enhancing Remote Follow-Up for Heart Failure Patients

AI's robust computational capabilities are proving invaluable across various clinical domains, including optimizing remote follow-up procedures. While CardioMEMS [86] has demonstrated efficacy in reducing heart failure re-hospitalizations by monitoring pulmonary artery hemodynamics, its invasiveness and cost constraints limit its widespread adoption for remote monitoring. A recent stride in this direction is showcased by the LINK-HF study [87], which explored non-invasive remote monitoring devices to track readmission rates in heart failure patients over 3 months. The study harnessed a chest sensor capable of recording physiological parameters, such as ECG waveforms, and generating clinical alerts when deviations from expected values occurred. Employing a machine learning algorithm to detect readmission risks, the study achieved sensitivity levels ranging from 76% to 88%, coupled with a specificity of 85%. Impressively, the median duration from initial alert to patient readmission was 6.5 days. This investigation underscores that wearable sensors augmented by machine learning exhibit predictive accuracy akin to previously reported implantable devices, offering added convenience and fewer clinically relevant complications.

In light of its distinct advantages, artificial intelligence effectively processes and categorizes data, yielding reliable insights that guide informed decisions and optimize clinical assistance. This, in turn, maximizes the utilization of human resources and ameliorates the challenge posed by clinical workforce shortages. The trajectory ahead suggests an escalating integration of AI into clinical practice. As AI progressively takes on the mantle of laborious manual tasks inherent in traditional clinical workflows, clinicians will remain at the forefront, steering the implementation of AI and the development of these algorithmic models.

## 3.4 Cardiomyopathy

Shao-Hua Guo and Kang-Yin Chen

Cardiomyopathy refers to the abnormal functioning and structural changes within the heart resulting from myocardial disease. This often manifests as tissue hypoperfusion, edema, fluid accumulation, and arrhythmias and involves various components of the pericardium and thoracic cavity. As per the classification by the American Heart Association (AHA) [88], cardiomyopathy can be categorized into primary and secondary forms. Primary cardiomyopathy primarily affects the heart muscle itself and includes hypertrophic, dilated, and restrictive types. Conversely, secondary cardiomyopathy involves myocardial infiltration as a manifestation of systemic ailments. Treatment approaches encompass heart failure staging, variable activity restriction, cardioverter-defibrillator implantation, and even heart transplantation for refractory cases. Despite recent strides in cardiovascular disease management, cardiomyopathy remains a significant contributor to cardiovascular mortality [89]. Notably, hypertrophic cardiomyopathy stands as a leading cause of sudden cardiac death among athletes, while diminished ejection fraction due to dilated cardiomyopathy often necessitates heart transplantation. Early recognition of cardiomyopathy is crucial, as it allows patients to receive prompt and standardized treatment. Subsequently, this can substantially diminish mortality and complications, potentially improving patients' prognosis. For instance, survival rates for patients with non-obstructive hypertrophic cardiomyopathy following surgical obstruction removal mirror those of the general population and surpass outcomes for patients without obstruction even after surgical intervention [90]. Echocardiography plays a vital role in cardiomyopathy diagnosis and assessment, but its high cost and technical demands make it unsuitable for population-wide screening, especially among asymptomatic individuals. ECGs, conversely, offer a cost-effective and widely accessible alternative. Recent efforts have explored the integration of AI into ECG-based automatic cardiomyopathy diagnosis. Multiple models and algorithms have demonstrated that AI-enhanced ECG analysis effectively detects and diagnoses cardiomyopathy with markedly improved accuracy compared to clinical experts. This section highlights the advancements in AI-driven ECG applications for cardiomyopathy diagnosis.

### 3.4.1 Dilated Cardiomyopathy

Shrivastava et al. [91], based at the Mayo Medical Center [92], retrained a model to differentiate patients with dilated cardiomyopathy and an ejection fraction ≤35% from healthy controls. This was an extension of a previously established CNN model that predicted dilated cardiomyopathy with an ejection fraction ≤45%. The outcomes indicated a sensitivity of 98.8% for diagnosing dilated cardiomyopathy in the entire cohort. The specificity was 44.8%, and the area under the receiver operating characteristic curve (AUC) was 0.955 (95% CI: 0.945–0.966). With a 1% prevalence of dilated cardiomyopathy, the model's positive predictive value was 1.8%, while the negative predictive value remained at 100%. At a 5% prevalence, the positive predictive value rose to 8.6%, and the negative predictive value remained high at 99.9%. Subgroup analyses revealed consistently high diagnostic efficacy of the AI-ECG model, with AUC values exceeding 0.9 across various conditions, except for the left bundle branch block. This study underscores the potential of AI-ECG as an accessible and cost-effective screening tool, particularly for at-risk individuals, including asymptomatic first-degree relatives. Beyond diagnosis, AI holds promise in identifying cardiomyopathy patients at risk. Gemell et al. [93] highlighted the challenge of identifying microfibrous tissue scars associated with dilated cardiomyopathy, often implicated in ventricular arrhythmia events and sudden death. Using vector electrocardiograms, they simulated different intracardiac scar patterns under varying pacing conditions, deriving indicators and evaluating changes to pinpoint scar presence, location, and size. Employing machine learning, they further enhanced scar localization for identifying high-risk arrhythmia patients. This approach offers a potential non-invasive means to address scar-related risks in dilated cardiomyopathy patients. In the field of genetic mutations, AI plays a pivotal role. Carriers of the phosphoprotein p.Arg14del gene mutation are at risk of developing dilated or arrhythmogenic cardiomyopathy, characterized by distinct electrocardiographic features [94]. A learning model was crafted by analyzing electrocardiograms from carriers of the p.Arg14del mutation and matched healthy controls by age and gender. The AI model exhibited exceptional sensitivity and accuracy in identifying the p.Arg14del mutation, outperforming cardiologists. Notably, T-wave patterns were identified as significant discriminators in this genetic context. This highlights AI's potential for precise genetic mutation detection in cardiomyopathy cases.

### 3.4.2 Hypertrophic Cardiomyopathy

In the domain of hypertrophic cardiomyopathy, the utilization of AI algorithms based on 12-lead ECG has proven significant. These algorithms can analyze the unique ECG characteristics of patients with hypertrophic cardiomyopathy, ultimately leading to the establishment of diagnostic models aimed at identifying this high-risk condition and reducing the risks of sudden death. Various AI techniques have been employed to diagnose and analyze hypertrophic cardiomyopathy. Rahman et al. [95], from Canada, employed a heartbeat classification approach on 12-lead ECG to identify hypertrophic cardiomyopathy. They utilized random forest and support vector machine algorithms to train and test the heartbeat classifier. By extracting 504 features from ECG signals to represent and classify heartbeats, the majority-classified subjects with hypertrophic cardiomyopathy were accurately diagnosed with a diagnostic accuracy of 0.94. This significantly outperformed conventional logistic regression. Ko's team [16], drawing from the Mayo Clinic electronic database, conducted extensive screening of hypertrophic cardiomyopathy patients and matched controls using convolutional neural networks (CNN) to train and validate a diagnostic model. This model achieved an AUC of 0.95 (95% CI: 0.94–0.97). Interestingly, postoperative recognition of hypertrophic cardiomyopathy decreased dramatically from 72% preoperatively to 2.5% in patients who underwent interventricular septal resection, indicating the model's sensitivity to post-surgical changes. Furthermore, this diagnostic model retained its effectiveness regardless of ECG findings of ventricular hypertrophy or the presence of myotome mutations, showing its robust clinical utility.

Notably, models for identifying hypertrophic cardiomyopathy have not only been established based on adult ECGs but have also shown effectiveness in adolescents and children. Siontis et al. [96] included a cohort of 300 hypertrophic cardiomyopathy patients and 18,439 controls, constructing a hypertrophic cardiomyopathy detection model based on the 12-lead ECG. This model achieved an impressive AUC of 0.98, with a positive predictive value of 22% and a negative predictive value of 99%. It is noteworthy that this model's accuracy extended across diverse demographics, including men, women, genotypically positive, and genotypically negative hypertrophic cardiomyopathy patients.

These findings collectively highlight the substantial effectiveness of current ECG-based AI models in diagnosing hypertrophic cardiomyopathy, demonstrating consistent accuracy across different ages, genders, and genetic phenotypes.

### 3.4.3 Myocardial Amyloidosis

AI-driven ECG analysis has also shown promise in detecting myocardial amyloidosis. Grogan et al. [97] developed a deep neural network model to predict myocardial amyloidosis in patients with light chain and transthyretin protein-related forms, comparing them to age- and gender-matched controls from Mayo Clinic records spanning 2000–2019. The model exhibited an impressive AUC of 0.91 and a positive predictive value of 0.86 for both types of myocardial amyloidosis. The AI model successfully predicted the presence of myocardial amyloidosis over six months before clinical diagnosis in 59% of cases. In this study, the V5 lead ECG test, with an AUC of 0.87 and an accuracy of 0.78, emerged as the best predictor among single lead models. Additionally, the limb lead model achieved an AUC of 0.90 with an accuracy of 0.85. This research underscores that AI-powered ECG models hold the potential to effectively detect myocardial amyloidosis, enabling early identification of this life-threatening condition. Moreover, combining

AI-driven ECG analysis with cardiac ultrasound can further enhance the diagnostic performance of the model [18]. This integration of additional data sources has the potential to improve the accuracy and reliability of myocardial amyloidosis detection, ultimately aiding in early diagnosis and improving patient outcomes.

### 3.4.4 Multi-disease Label Model

A pioneering approach involves the creation of a multi-disease label model, as demonstrated by Adam et al. [98]. This study harnessed a novel discrete wavelet transform technique in conjunction with nonlinear features to automatically characterize ECG signals for differentiation among various cardiovascular diseases. The diseases encompassed hypertrophic cardiomyopathy, dilated cardiomyopathy, and myocardial infarction and included healthy individuals as controls. Notably, four nonlinear features—fuzzy entropy, sample entropy, fractal dimension, and signal energy—were extracted from wavelet transform coefficients. These features were subjected to sequence forward selection (SFS) and subsequently sorted using the Relief method. The top 15 ranked features, as determined by the Relief method, were employed in a K-nearest neighbor classifier. Remarkably, this approach achieved a maximum classification accuracy of 99.27%, sensitivity of 99.74%, and specificity of 98.08%. This method can expedite and enhance clinicians' ability to diagnose cardiovascular diseases with heightened accuracy. Incorporating a combination of deep learning and machine learning techniques, Tison et al. [17] pursued a comprehensive strategy. Rather than opting for an end-to-end deep learning architecture, the authors derived a feature vector from the deep learning model and integrated it into a machine learning framework encompassing 35,446 ECG sets. The aim was to predict conditions like pulmonary hypertension, hypertrophic cardiomyopathy, amyloidosis, and mitral valve prolapse. A satisfactory predictive performance was achieved, although some variations were present in the diagnostic accuracy across different conditions. While the AUC for predicting mitral valve prolapse was comparatively low valued at 0.78, the detection of hypertrophic cardiomyopathy yielded a higher AUC of 0.91. This study underscores the potential of combining deep learning and machine learning for multi-disease diagnosis, despite varying levels of accuracy for different conditions.

### 3.4.5 Summary

In the field of cardiomyopathy diagnosis and classification, the integration of AI with ECG analysis has yielded promising outcomes. Current research and model development have demonstrated notable levels of accuracy, often surpassing those of clinical ECG experts. Nonetheless, these studies encounter certain limitations, highlighting a gap between theoretical advancements and practical clinical implementation. One key limitation involves the establishment and validation of models, which typically rely on distinct cohorts of cardiomyopathy patients and healthy controls. In real-world clinical scenarios, the spectrum of disease types is far broader. For instance, it remains uncertain whether an algorithm designed to identify dilated cardiomyopathy can effectively differentiate it from ventricular dilation caused by ischemic cardiomyopathy within a diverse population. Similarly, the hypertrophic cardiomyopathy model's ability to distinguish between hypertrophic cardiomyopathy and hypertensive left ventricular hypertrophy across a wide range of individuals requires validation for model stability within a broader context. Another challenge stems from the inherent "black box" nature of AI methodologies. Despite the proliferation of various models and algorithms, the precise ECG features that correlate with specific diseases remain inadequately understood and defined. The lack of transparency in AI-ECG diagnosis hinders a comprehensive understanding of the underlying mechanisms, necessitating further exploration and refinement.

## 3.5 Hereditary Arrhythmia and AI-ECG Applications

Wen-Hua Song, Tong Liu, and Jia-Wei Xie

Advancements in genetic testing for inherited heart diseases have progressed rapidly over the last two decades. With the increase in disease-causing genes and their variants, the diagnosis and understanding of inherited heart diseases have become more complex. Pathogenic variants often exhibit atypical externalities or manifest later in life, leading to delayed diagnosis. Genetic background, environmental factors, and lifestyle choices further complicate clinical presentation and treatment timing. Some genetic disorders, such as prolonged QT interval or cardiac hypertrophy, can be diagnosed based on clinical signs. However, sudden cardiac death (SCD) in young patients might be the only indication in related families, and current genetic tests can only identify potentially causative variants or mutations of uncertain significance.

This review aims to focus on the latest developments in AI-ECG for genetic arrhythmias, specifically congenital long QT syndrome, Brugada syndrome, and catecholaminergic polymorphic ventricular tachycardia. The objective is to provide clinicians with insights into the evolving trends in this field.

### 3.5.1 AI and Machine Learning

Machine learning is a pivotal aspect of AI research, primarily concerned with building computational models through data-driven learning, especially in sample classification. Over the years, various machine learning methods have emerged, from support vector machines in the 1990s to random forests in the early 2000s. Recent advances in data sources, digitization, and data collection have significantly expanded the application of these algorithms. Machine learning has found applications in diverse fields, such as using eye movements for subject verification and classifying aquatic animals to assess water quality. Clinical medicine is a particularly prominent domain for machine learning, facilitating personalized medicine, medical imaging, and disease diagnosis [99, 100].

### 3.5.2 Application of AI in QT Interval Measurement

The QT interval in an ECG signifies the duration of the cardiomyocyte action potential, dependent on the balance between inward and outward currents. AP consists of five stages: the polar phase (stage 0), initial rapid repolarization (stage 1), plateau phase (stage 2), late rapid repolarization (stage 3), and resting phase (stage 4). The European Society of Cardiology guidelines suggest a normal QT interval between 360 ms and 480 ms for both genders. AI algorithms can simulate human ECG interpretation, mimicking cardiologist knowledge to identify heart rate, P-waves before QRS complexes, and pathological waveform changes [101–103].

John R. Giudicessi et al. [26] introduced an AI-based algorithm to determine QTc intervals. They employed a deep neural network trained on 1.6 million 12-lead ECGs from over half a million patients. The algorithm predicted QTc intervals with high accuracy, validated against measurements taken by cardiologists. This application provides a cost-effective and efficient means of screening for congenital long QT syndrome. Additionally, a natural language processor (NLP) was developed to identify prolonged QT intervals more efficiently than conventional ECG machines, enhancing diagnostic accuracy.

### 3.5.3 Application of Machine Learning in Genetic Arrhythmias

#### 3.5.3.1 Congenital Long QT Syndrome (LQTS)

LQTS is a primary ECG disorder characterized by an increased risk of SCD due to malignant ventricular arrhythmias [104]. This syndrome can arise from congenital ion channel mutations or acquired factors, resulting in a prolonged ECG QT interval that is ≥450 ms.

##### Discovery of LQTS

The first identification of LQTS occurred in 1957 through the work of Jervell and Lange-Nielsen (JLN). They observed a family where parents exhibited normal QT intervals and hearing, while their six children displayed varied characteristics. Four children had both prolonged QT intervals and congenital sensorineural deafness, and three of them experienced sudden death. Subsequent investigation confirmed autosomal recessive inheritance for JLN syndrome. In the 1960s, Romano and Ward separately reported cases of prolonged QT intervals with normal hearing, indicating autosomal dominant inheritance.

##### Genetic Background of LQTS

LQTS arises from alterations in repolarization or depolarization currents. There are currently 13 recognized genetic subtypes. Various types of mutations affecting potassium ($K^+$) channels lead to LQTS subtypes: type 1 (KCNQ1), type 2 (KCNH2), type 5 (KCNE1), type 6 (KCNE2), type 7 (KCNJ2), and type 13 (KCNJ5). Sodium (Na+) channel mutations cause LQTS3 (SCN5A) and LQTS10 (SCN4B) due to functional gain. LQTS8 (CACNA1C), known as Timothy syndrome, involves L-type calcium ($Ca^{2+}$) channels. Other genetic mutations contribute to LQTS4

(ANKB), LQTS9 (CAV3), LQTS11 (AKAP9), and LQTS12 (SNTA1). Additionally, long QT intervals are associated with sudden death in epilepsy, where neuronal $Na^+$ channel subtypes lead to the amplification of late $Na^+$ current (Ina, L) [105, 106].

#### Application of AI-ECG in Congenital Long QT Syndrome (LQTS)

In a study on congenital LQTS, Gary Tse et al. [107] applied the random survival forest algorithm, the so-called random survival forest algorithm, which is a random forest method for the analysis of right-censored survival data. The researchers introduced a new survival splitting rule for growing survival trees and a new missing data algorithm for imputing missing data. The researchers included clinical data of patients diagnosed with LQTS from 1997 to 2019, explored important risk factors for ventricular arrhythmias in this cohort, and compared the performance of traditional Cox regression and random survival forest. In this study, RSF constructs hundreds of trees, and randomization is introduced in two forms: randomly drawn data-guided samples for growing trees, and node splits on randomly selected predictors for growing tree learners.

Compared with the Cox proportional hazards model, RSF showed clear advantages. The algorithm makes no assumptions about individual hazard functions and ranks the importance of spontaneous VT/VF predictors. The boosting tree structure in RSF can capture the nonlinear effects and complex interactions between variables, which can reduce the prediction variance and deviation and significantly improve the calculation accuracy. In addition, RSF can handle the effects of interventions and predictors, whereas traditional methods using Cox or Kaplan-Meier analyses exploit linear combinations of attributes. The study found that, in addition to predicting mortality in heart failure patients receiving cardiac resynchronization therapy, RSF can be used to improve the prediction of all-cause mortality in heart failure, heart failure-related hospitalization events, and costs. Furthermore, the model successfully predicted in-hospital mortality in patients with cardiac arrest in the intensive care unit, as well as all-cause mortality in patients who acquired LQTS. This study is the first to demonstrate that the RSF model can significantly improve the VT/VF predictive value of LQTS.

### 3.5.3.2 Brugada Syndrome (BrS)

#### Discovery of BrS

The three Brugada brothers from Spain made a special report at the annual meeting of the North American Society for Cardiac Pacing and Electrophysiology (NASPE) in 1991. Later, they summarized another four cases and published a paper in the *Journal of the American Heart Association* (AHA) in 1992, which was titled "Right bundle-branch block and ST-segment elevation in leads V1 through V3: A marker for sudden death in patients without demonstrable structural heart disease." Once the paper was published, it immediately attracted the attention of doctors from all over the world. After reporting many similar cases, Professor Yan Ganxin from the United States named it "Brugada syndrome" for the first time.

### Genetic Background of BrS

In 1998, American scholar Chen et al. used PCR-SSCP analysis, DNA sequence determination, and other molecular biology experimental techniques to find that each of the three BrS individuals carried the SCN5A gene mutation on one allele and then proved that BrS was an "ionic ion" at the molecular level, channel structure defect disease, and is an autosomal dominant genetic disease. Scholars from various countries subsequently discovered dozens of different sites and types of SCNSA gene mutations.

### Application of AI-ECG in Brugada Syndrome (BrS)

BrS is a cardiac disease with a high risk of ventricular tachycardia/ventricular fibrillation (VT/VF) and SCD. Clinical symptoms, ECG markers, and invasive tests such as electrophysiological studies can be used for risk stratification but are difficult to predict, especially in asymptomatic patients. In previous studies, most ECG-related data were measured manually, and there were inevitable subjective biases. Automated measurements have not been used for risk prediction and may provide information that is difficult to obtain with manual measurements.

Gary Tse et al. [108] investigated further on BrS-related predictors; they retrospectively analyzed BrS patients who were treated in the same tertiary hospital from 2000 to 2018. The parameters related to P, Q, R, S, and T waves are automatically extracted by machine, including 12-lead ECG vector value, electric axis, amplitude, duration, etc. The primary endpoint was spontaneous ventricular tachycardia/fibrillation (VT/VF) events during follow-up. The investigators first identified ECG variables that were significantly predictive of the primary endpoint by Cox regression and then generated a simple algorithm based on a decision tree learning approach, a risk stratification scoring system. Automated ECG measurements related to depolarization and repolarization are helpful for risk stratification of BrS patients, the results showed.

In another Hong Kong cohort study [109], Cox regression was also used to identify significant risk predictors of BrS. Non-linear interactions between variables were extracted by non-negative matrix factorization (NMF) and incorporated into the RSF model. The advantage of RSF is that it can capture the nonlinear effects and complex interactions between variables, thereby reducing the prediction variance and bias and improving the predictive performance of left ventricular structure predictors for cardiac arrest events and LQTS ventricular arrhythmia events. In summary, machine learning technology reduces the interference of human factors and subjective bias and significantly improves the overall risk stratification efficiency of BrS.

## 3.5.3.3 Catecholaminergic Polymorphic Ventricular Tachycardia (CPVT)

### Discovery of CPVT

The first reported case of catecholaminergic polymorphic ventricular tachycardia (CPVT) was documented by Reid in 1975, and it was systematically described by Coumel in 1978.

**Genetic Background of CPVT**
CPVT has distinct genetic underpinnings. It is divided into two clinical categories based on different pathogenic genes, namely, CPVT1 and CPVT2. CPVT1 is inherited in an autosomal dominant manner and is caused by mutations in the RyR2 gene within cardiomyocytes. Around 50% of CPVT patients have RyR2 gene mutations. CPVT2, on the other hand, follows autosomal recessive inheritance and is less common than CPVT1. It is linked to mutations in the CASQ2 gene (cardiomyocyte calcium-storage protein), accounting for approximately 1–2% of cases. Overall, approximately 60% of CPVT patients can be identified with mutations in the RyR2 or CASQ2 genes.

**Application of AI-ECG in CPVT**
Martti Juhola et al. [110] proposed an innovative diagnostic approach for hereditary heart diseases, specifically in patients with a familial history of SCD or those with nonspecific clinical features. The approach involves utilizing human-induced pluripotent stem cell-derived cardiomyocytes (IPSC-CMS) as a diagnostic tool. This model enables the study of disease pathophysiology, treatment, and diagnosis. The researchers focused on detecting potential hereditary heart diseases using the calcium signals of cells derived from IPSC-CMS. By employing machine learning methods, they created a calcium transient map that allowed them to identify abnormal calcium transients associated with different heart disorders. This study aimed to distinguish between CPVT, long QT syndrome (LQT), and hypertrophic cardiomyopathy (HCM) based on these Ca2+ transients. The results were promising, demonstrating a high classification accuracy of up to 87% for these three disorders. The machine learning approach effectively identified disease-specific characteristics of Ca2+ transients. Even when incorporating healthy controls into the classification, the accuracy remained high at approximately 79%. This indicates the potential of machine learning as a powerful tool for accurately classifying IPSC-CMS and suggests its potential as a future diagnostic method. The researchers also noted that as more advanced methods, such as differentiating blood cells directly into cardiomyocytes, emerge in the future, diagnostic tools for inherited heart diseases are likely to become more diverse and effective.

### 3.5.4 Summary and Prospects

Machine learning, a computer algorithm capable of learning complex patterns from data, holds significant potential for medical advancements. Many diagnostic and management decisions in healthcare rely on digital information from individual patients, such as ECG and echocardiography. With the exponential growth of clinical records, wearable devices, sensor data, and medical imaging, the complexity of medical practice has surpassed the capacity of the human mind. This has led to variations in knowledge, skills, and practices among different clinicians. Machine learning algorithms, when appropriately designed, validated, and implemented, can play a crucial role in capturing, interpreting, and synthesizing medical data from diverse sources. These algorithms can provide comprehensive insights to clinicians, enabling them to offer informed guidance and assistance to patients in various clinical scenarios.

Accurately predicting the impact of newly identified genetic variants on disease risk remains a challenge in contemporary clinical genetics. While several tools have been developed to predict the effects of common genetic variants and assess their likelihood of causing disease, machine learning approaches are still not precise enough in some cases. These approaches may overlook important parameters that define the relationship between target genes and disease outcomes, such as distinguishing between gain-of-function and loss-of-function variants. As a result, there is a need for further research and high-quality studies to explore the application of AI-ECG in hereditary arrhythmias. The use of machine learning in this context could potentially enhance our understanding of genetic influences on arrhythmias and lead to more accurate predictions of disease risks.

## 3.6 Ventricular Arrhythmias

Hui-Min Chu and Guo-Hua Fu

Ventricular arrhythmia (VA) is a type of abnormal heart rhythm disorder that includes a range of conditions, including pre-ventricular systole, ventricular tachycardia, ventricular flutter, and atrial fibrillation. VAs can lead to hemodynamic instability and stand as a primary driver of sudden cardiac death. Timely and precise identification, as well as effective management of these arrhythmias, hold crucial importance in preventing cardiovascular mortality. Variability arises in human interpretation of VAs and ECG readings depending on the level of professional expertise. The integration of AI in ECG analysis exhibits the potential to enhance diagnostic accuracy and operational efficiency.

### 3.6.1 Integration of AI for VA Recognition

In initial studies, AI technology was predominantly applied to automating arrhythmia classification [111]. The process involves ECG data collection, data processing, segmentation, and feature extraction, culminating in the development and testing of a data classification model suitable for clinical applications [111]. However, disparities in target disease detection and performance are evident among published AI arrhythmia classification models. These differences arise from factors like ECG data collection methods (single lead or multi-lead), signal processing techniques, feature extraction methodologies, and utilization of diverse machine learning models. Currently, established arrhythmia databases adhering to global standards, such as MIT-BIH, EDB, CU, and NST5, rely on data from two ECG leads [111]. Drawing from research results utilizing the aforementioned databases, different ECG feature extraction techniques (e.g., RR intervals, wavelet transformations, morphological features, random speculation methods, etc.) and distinct machine learning models (e.g., weighted linear regression, weighted support vector machine, logistic regression) yield identification accuracies for VAs ranging from 83% to 97%, sensitivities of 80–91%, and specificities of 85–99% [112–119]. The substantial heterogeneity across these study outcomes underscores the need for comprehensive refinement to achieve more consistent and precise VA classifications. Moreover, the research suggests that thoracic lead V1-V2 offers optimal suitability for VA identification and classification, with a recommended combination of limb lead II and thoracic lead V2 potentially yielding improved model recognition outcomes.

Derived from the MIT-BIH database, Mathews et al. [120] conducted an investigation employing a low-frequency sampling rate of 114 Hz. They harnessed a deep learning model to discern ventricular ectopic rhythm and supraventricular ectopic rhythm using single-lead ECG data. The study employed two specific machine learning methods: the restricted Boltzmann machine (RBM) and the deep belief network (DBN). However, while trained on single-lead ECG data, the resulting model exhibited an average recognition accuracy of 93.63% for ventricular ectopic rhythm, which was deemed less than satisfactory.

Zheng et al. [121], in their 2020 publication, introduced a novel feature extraction algorithm. This algorithm transformed one-dimensional ECG data into a two-dimensional format for enhanced processing. The study incorporated a substantial dataset of 40,258 12-lead ECG records. From this dataset, 3332 optimal feature parameters were extracted. A range of machine learning models underwent training and testing, culminating in the selection of the optimal classification models—the extreme gradient boosting tree model (EG-BT) and the gradient boosting tree model (GBT). Remarkable results were generated by employing the MIT-BIH database for model testing. The model achieved a balanced accuracy F1 score of 98.6% for VA recognition, with a positive prediction accuracy of 98.0% and an impressive sensitivity of 99.1%. This outcome is highly promising, suggesting that the combination of the feature extraction algorithm alongside the extreme gradient boosting tree model or gradient boosting tree model might represent the optimal approach for VA recognition.

### 3.6.2 AI in VA Origin Localization

While an array of references and literature address the localization of VA, most studies tend to rely on small sample sizes and only focus on specific subtypes of these arrhythmias. However, these findings have not been translated into a real-life practical setting. Current electrophysiologists continue to rely on traditional learning, memory, and experience. AI technology holds the potential to leverage extensive datasets for deep exploration of hidden features. By doing so, it can achieve precise localization of VAs, ultimately resulting in algorithmic solutions applicable in real-world scenarios. Subsequently, this may aid surgeons in swiftly and effectively conducting high-quality surgeries, thereby diminishing complications and risks for patients.

Nakamura et al. [122] sought to enhance the precision of existing algorithms for pinpointing the site of origin of ventricular precontraction by incorporating two distinct machine learning models—the support vector machine (SVM) and convolutional neural network (CNN). In this study, a total of 116 pre-ventricular systole samples were collected from 111 patients. The two machine learning models were trained and evaluated using 12-lead ECG data. Pre-ventricular systole locations were categorized into four groups, namely, right ventricular outflow tract, left ventricular outflow tract, right ventricular non-outflow tract, and left ventricular non-outflow tract. The study compared the predictive accuracy of the two models in determining whether the origin of pre-ventricular systole was in the left or right ventricle. The average weighted accuracy for the four pre-ventricular contraction localization categories was 0.85, 0.80, 0.73, and 0.86 for SVM, CNN, electrophysiological experts, and existing algorithms, respectively. Additionally, the machine learning model's F1 scores for positive prediction accuracy, sensitivity, and balanced accuracy outperformed those of medical experts, exhibiting comparability to existing algorithms. Among the two models, SVM demonstrated superior accuracy in predicting the four types of pre-ventricular contractions of 0.94, 0.87, 0.79, and 0.90, respectively, surpassing CNN. Despite the machine learning model's improved accuracy compared to electrophysiology experts, it fell short of surpassing the performance of existing algorithms.

In a study by He et al. [123], artificial intelligence was employed to determine the origin of ventricular precontraction throughout the entire ventricle. In this study, 249 patients with ventricular pre-systole were selected. A novel algorithm was developed to automatically extract ventricular pre-systole instances from long-term 12-lead ECG data. These instances were then categorized and labeled into 374 sample groups, each containing multiple ventricular pre-systole data points. The database was divided into 11 categories based on the origin of ventricular pre-systole across the entire ventricle: left ventricular outflow tract, right ventricular outflow tract, left ventricular anterior wall base, left ventricular anterior wall middle, septal base, septal middle, left ventricular lower wall base, left ventricular lower wall middle, epicardium, right ventricular lower wall, and right ventricular anterior wall. Approximately 70% ($n = 257$) of the sample group data were used for training four distinct machine learning models: SVM, random forest (RF), gradient boosting decision tree (GBDT), and Gaussian Naive Bayes (GNB). The remaining 30% (n = 117) of the sample group data was reserved for model testing. The results indicated that the machine learning models achieved recognition accuracy, sensitivity, and specificity of 97.6%, 98.3%, and 96.7%, respectively, for VA detection. The machine learning model's accuracy in locating the origin of pre-ventricular systole ranged from 70.7% to 74.7%. When combined with adjacent region information, the accuracy was elevated to a range of 91.5–93.2%. These findings underscore that there is still significant room for improvement in enhancing the accuracy of machine learning models for precise localization of pre-ventricular contractions.

Professor Hui-Min Chu and his team at Ningbo First Hospital utilized the aforementioned feature extraction algorithm to extract 12-lead ECG data from patients who underwent successful catheter ablation surgery for outflow tract origin VAs and were definitively diagnosed by the team. They further subdivided the left and right ventricular outflow tract regions into specific subregions. These subdivisions included the left coronary sinus (LCC), right coronary sinus (RCC), ancillary coronary sinus (NCC), aorto-mitral ring junction (AMC), top of the left ventricle, and the junction of the left and right coronary sinuses for the left ventricular outflow tract. For the right ventricular outflow tract, the subdivisions comprised the anterior pulmonary sinus (AC), left sinus (AC), right sinus (RC), anterior septum, posterior septum, free wall, and other segments. The acquired ECG data was automatically categorized into these 13 regions. The patient's 12-lead standard ECGs taken prior to catheter ablation, which included QRS complexes during sinus rhythm and one QRS complex during VA, were used as input for building the database and training the machine learning model [124].

Building upon previous research findings, the team opted for the GBT to forecast the origin of the left and right ventricular outflow tract in cases of idiopathic VAs [125]. This study encompassed a cohort of 420 patients with outflow tract origin VAs, all of whom had undergone successful catheter ablation under the guidance of Professor Hui-Min Chu team. The patient cohort was divided into distinct groups: training, evaluation, and test groups. The machine learning model was trained on the training group and subsequently subjected to a black box test on the test group. The outcomes were then compared with predictions made by electrophysiologists before catheter ablation procedures. The findings revealed that the machine learning model exhibited exceptional performance on the test group, achieving an accuracy exceeding 97%, a remarkable feature Area Under the Curve (AUC) of 98.99%, a sensitivity of 96.97%, and a specificity of 100%. Notably, both accuracy and specificity surpassed human expert predictions, which stood at 94.29% and 81.72%, respectively. However, the sensitivity was on par with human experts valued at 97.86%. Furthermore, the machine learning model identified 1352 out of 1,600,800 automatically computed ECG variables that played a significant role in discerning the left and right ventricular outflow tract. Among these, three parameters associated with the V1 and V3 leads demonstrated great significance. To corroborate, the machine learning model scrutinized 155,784 ECG morphological characteristics and their deformations, discovering that 1003 variables held significant influence in predicting the left and right ventricular outflow tract. The three most pivotal parameters were the ratio of R-wave amplitude of lead III to that of V1 during VA, the ratio of R-wave amplitude of V2 lead in sinus rhythm to that of V3 lead during VA, and the ratio of R-wave amplitude of lead aVL in sinus rhythm to that of V1 lead during VA. These findings hold promising potential for clinical applications. Concurrently, a comparative assessment of 12 existing studies focused on left and right ventricular outflow tract prediction indicated a lack of robust universality across these studies. This underscores the importance of pursuing strong generality in machine learning models, which remains a pivotal direction for advancements in the field of artificial intelligence.

### 3.6.3 AI in Ventricular Tachycardia and Ventricular Fibrillation Identification

In clinical practice, distinguishing between ventricular fibrillation and ventricular tachycardia often relies on doctors' clinical experience, which can introduce subjectivity and potentially result in misdiagnosis and harm to patients. Thus, there is a growing interest in leveraging AI for the accurate differentiation of these arrhythmias.

Alwan et al. [126] underscored the limitations of existing machine learning models in discerning arrhythmias, particularly due to the low-dimensional nature of ECG signals. While these models could identify VAs, they struggled to distinguish between ventricular tachycardia and ventricular fibrillation. To address this, the study introduced high-dimensional feature vectors in capturing ECG signals and employed data from the AHA, CU, and MIT-BIH databases to categorize arrhythmias into ventricular tachyarrhythmia, ventricular fibrillation, and other rhythm types. Results demonstrated that the utilization of high-dimensional eigenvector techniques enhanced the ability of the machine learning model to differentiate between ventricular tachycardia and ventricular fibrillation. However, it exhibited reduced sensitivity to other heart rhythms. These findings suggest that an effective approach may involve combining the strengths of diverse feature spaces to enhance the recognition and discrimination capabilities of machine learning models. By doing so, AI could offer valuable insights and contribute to more precise identification of ventricular tachycardia and ventricular fibrillation, ultimately leading to improved patient care and diagnosis accuracy.

Mjahad et al. [127] undertook a study employing data from the AHA and MIT-BIH databases to enhance accuracy and minimize information loss during ECG feature selection and model training stages. They integrated time-frequency (t-f) compensation image techniques to mitigate data loss. Four distinct machine learning models were trained, including L2-adjusted logistic regression (L2RLR), adaptive neural network classifiers (ANNC), SVM, and bag classifiers (BAGG). The findings revealed that ANNC and BAGG outperformed the other models. For the detection of ventricular fibrillation, including short bouts, ANNC achieved an accuracy of 95.56% and sensitivity of 95.56%, while BAGG reached an accuracy of 98.46% and sensitivity of 98.46%. Both models demonstrated a high specificity of 98.80% and 98.43%, respectively. Regarding ventricular tachycardia detection, ANNC achieved an accuracy of 98.87% with a sensitivity of 88.80% and specificity of 99.52%. BAGG's performance was also notable, with an accuracy of 98.82%, sensitivity of 84.58%, and remarkable specificity of 99.86%. Furthermore, the study performed a statistical analysis of existing machine learning models utilizing AHA, CU, and MIT-BIH data for detecting ventricular fibrillation and ventricular tachycardia. For ventricular tachycardia detection, only four models were employed, achieving accuracies ranging from 48.0% to 92.0%, with sensitivity and specificity details not provided. In contrast, ventricular fibrillation detection involved 12 models, with accuracy ranging from 86.6% to 100%, sensitivity ranging from 90.47% to 98.15%, and specificity ranging from 88.00% to 97.03%. The study suggests that incorporating t-f compensation image technology into machine learning models can yield improved performance, further enhancing ventricular fibrillation and ventricular tachycardia recognition rates. This advancement holds the potential to significantly reduce the substantial harm stemming from clinical misdiagnoses, ultimately benefiting patients' well-being.

The timely application of automated external defibrillators (AEDs) during out-of-hospital cardiac arrest (OHCA) is crucial, but accurately determining whether an electric shock is needed remains a challenge. Picon et al. [128] devised a solution by employing CNN and long short-term memory (LSTM) networks for deep learning. This approach aids in identifying occurrences of ventricular fibrillation and facilitating decision-making for AEDs. Two databases were included in this study: (1) the public database, the ambulate ECG data of patients with arrhythmia for the first time and (2) monitor data recorded after cardiac arrest in OHCA patients. The algorithm also takes into account balance accuracy (BAC), unweighted average sensitivity (Se), and specificity (Sp). The results showed that the BAC, Se, and Sp of ventricular fibrillation are identified as 99.3%, 99.7%, and 98.9% in a public database, while in the OHCA database, they are identified as 98.0%, 96.7%, and 96.7%, respectively.

### 3.6.4 AI in Predicting VAs

The prediction of VAs holds the potential for reducing sudden death rates associated with various heart diseases. Okada et al. [129] introduced a novel machine learning approach to analyze late gadolinium enhancement cardiac magnetic resonance (LGE-CMR) images, aiming to derive stromal space complexity (SSC) for predicting VA occurrences in patients with ischemic cardiomyopathy. In this study, a cohort of 122 patients diagnosed with ischemic cardiomyopathy and EF $\leq$ 35% who had no history of previous VA underwent LGE-CMR imaging. Utilizing three-dimensional reconstruction of the left ventricle, a machine learning statistical algorithm was applied to analyze signal intensity within the images, leading to the extraction of SSC and calculation of complexity scores (CS). Over a follow-up period of five years, 40 patients experienced VA events, and the machine learning algorithm demonstrated an accuracy of 81% in predicting VA occurrences. Notably, patients who experienced VA exhibited significantly higher CS values compared to those without VA ($0.5 \pm 0.5$ vs. $0.1 \pm 0.2$, $P < 0.001$). Multivariate Cox regression analysis highlighted CS as an independent predictor of VA events (HR 1.5, 95% CI: 1.2–2.0, $P = 0.002$). This study showcases the potential of SSC analysis in clarifying the risk of VAs among patients with ischemic cardiomyopathy. The application of this approach, particularly in identifying low-risk VA cases, offers promising insights for risk assessment and intervention strategies to mitigate the occurrence of VAs and associated complications.

Bhattacharya et al. [130] used machine learning algorithms to scrutinize clinical data, aiming to identify predictors of VAs in patients with hypertrophic cardiomyopathy. Their study included a cohort of 711 patients, among whom 61 had a history of ventricular tachycardia or ventricular fibrillation. By extracting pertinent clinical variables, the researchers trained and tested a machine learning model through sampling. An evaluation of 93 clinical variables was conducted, leading to the selection of 22 variables that emerged as potential predictors. The machine learning approach was then employed to discern 12 predictors of VA. The culmination of these efforts yielded the creation of an HCM-VAr-Risk model, boasting a sensitivity of 0.73, a specificity of 0.76, and a C-index of 0.83. Importantly, this model demonstrated superior predictive capacity for VA compared to the guidelines provided by the

European Society of Cardiology and the American College of Cardiology, thereby positioning it as a recommended predictive tool.

### 3.6.5 Future Outlook

The accuracy and convenience of machine learning models allow for AI application in VA in the future. For example, in the recognition of VAs, machine learning models should be adapted to single-lead ECG, increasing its usability. At present, the origin location prediction model of VA is also more used in the left and right ventricular outflow tract area, and the whole ventricular origin location should also be the future direction of AI, and the current research shows that some research models do not have good universality, which limits the accessibility of AI. In addition, clinical usage of AI models should be adapted for real-life circumstances. For example, although SVM models in novel studies have obtained good results, the model is costly and has low practicability, thus it is not suitable for clinical work. At present, there is still a lack of algorithms that can be applied in clinical practice. It is believed that with the development of technology and the deepening of clinical practice research, more accurate AI will be used for clinical identification of VAs, locating the origin of ventricular pre-systole, distinguishing ventricular tachycardia from ventricular flutter, ventricular fibrillation, and predicting the occurrence of VAs, which will greatly improve the work efficiency and diagnostic accuracy of clinicians and electrophysiologists. It can help more patients identify and prevent the occurrence of malignant VAs and reduce the risk of sudden cardiac death.

## 3.7 Cardiac Pacing

Ni-Xiao Zhang and Tong Liu

AI research in the medical field is developing rapidly and has been widely used in various fields of medicine, including oncology, imaging, cardiology, various surgical procedures, and rehabilitation treatment [131]. The China Cardiovascular Diseases Report 2018 points out [132] that cardiovascular diseases currently account for the first place in the total causes of death of urban and rural residents, accounting for more than 40% of the death composition of residents. The total inpatient cost of cardiovascular and cerebrovascular diseases is also rapidly increasing. China's cardiovascular disease burden is increasing day by day and affecting public health. Therefore, it is of great significance to use efficient and cutting-edge technological means for cardiovascular prevention and control, medical cost reduction, and diagnosis and treatment effect improvement. At present, ECG intelligent diagnosis, cardiovascular imaging intelligent analysis, and cardiovascular disease screening have been carried out at home and abroad. This section aims to explore the application of AI technology in the field of cardiac pacing.

### 3.7.1 Overview of Cardiovascular AI

AI and machine learning are general terms for a group of algorithms that allow computers to discover patterns from data and make decisions [133]. The current technical means of implementing AI are mainly machine learning. Machine learning is the method of learning (or "guessing") general rules from limited observational data and applying those rules to unobserved samples. Traditional machine learning data processing processes include data pre-processing, feature extraction, feature transformation, and prediction [131]. For example, in supervised learning, researchers take clinical data, such as age, gender, blood pressure, blood lipid, myocardial enzyme profile, ECG index, and gene sequence. Along with basic sample data, the use of artificial neural networks, decision trees, support vector machines, naive Bayes, and other algorithms in machine learning can be integrated to build a prediction model for cardiovascular, all-cause, and other outcome events. Finally, we can evaluate the risk of other patients' outcome events through this model and provide guidance for clinical diagnosis and treatment. The construction of such supervised learning models must be based on large datasets, which is time-consuming and requires continuous training to improve its prediction accuracy [131]. However, rather than identifying predictors of outcome events, unsupervised approaches group similar patients by multiple characteristics, analyze the characteristics of individuals between similar groups, and correlate them with outcomes or treatment responses, i.e., attempt to identify new disease-causing mechanisms, genotypes, or phenotypes from the information hidden by the data [131]. In unsupervised learning, the goal is to uncover the information hidden in the data without human feedback.

### 3.7.2 AI and Cardiac Pacing Therapy

#### 3.7.2.1 AI's Application in Selecting Candidates for CRT Placement

Multiple clinical trials have shown that cardiac resynchronization therapy (CRT) can reduce morbidity and mortality in patients with heart failure [134]. However, although all patients meet the criteria for implantation, approximately 30% of patients do not respond to CRT treatment [21]. One application area for population classification based on unsupervised learning is to screen patients with higher precision who are suitable for CRT. One study [135] included 1106 patients with CRT and extracted 50 baseline data including epidemiologic data, serological tests, ECG, echocardiography, medication, and center of visit. These patients were divided into four groups by unsupervised learning. There were significant differences between the four groups in most clinical baselines and primary endpoint events, with two groups having a better response to CRT, a higher proportion of known predictors of CRT response, and a reduced risk of primary endpoint events. Combined with some novel ultrasound indicators, such as local longitudinal strain signal, CRT patients can be divided into five groups; the reactivity of the first group of patients is 50% and the reactivity of the fifth group is 92.7%. Interestingly, the first type of CRT patients had the lowest risk of event-free survival compared with other types of patients [136]. By extracting 28 indicators from 193 patients with CRT, Galli et al. divided the patients into two categories by the unsupervised learning method. The CRT response rate of the first type of patients was 89%, the CRT response rate of the second type was 34%, and the event-free survival rate of the latter was lower [137]. The inclusion criteria of CRT patients mainly depended on QRS duration and QRS form, and a certain proportion of non-response rate suggested that screening based on these two indicators had certain limitations. Therefore, Feeny et al. used an unsupervised learning method to divide 946 CRT patients into two categories based on ECG waveform, and the composite endpoints and LVEF improvement of the two groups were significantly different, and the results were not affected by QRS ≥ 150 ms and complete left bundle branch block (LBBB) [22]. These results suggest that unsupervised learning integrating multiple clinical parameters can distinguish between populations that respond well or poorly to CRT according to a pre-set number of categories, although differences in the parameters included may affect the final number of classifications.

The machine learning model predicted better responses to CRT than the traditional model of CRT reactivity. In one study, Kalscheur et al. compared the prediction effect of the random forest algorithm model with the traditional CRT prediction model. The findings of the study found that the prediction effect of the machine learning model was better than that of the model constructed by the bundle branch block pattern combined with QRS duration for the risk of all-cause death or hospitalization for heart failure 12 months after CRT. The risk of all-cause death or hospitalization for heart failure in the high-risk population screened by the random forest model was 8 times that of the low-risk population (HR 7.96) [138]. Feeny et al. included 925 patients with CRT to study the predictive model of CRT reactivity, defined as an increase of ≥10% in LVEF. The results showed that naive Bayes was the optimal machine learning model, and the prediction effect of this model was superior to the guidelines. Nine important variables were selected, including QRS morphology, QRS duration, New York Heart Association classification (NYHA), LVEF, left ventricular end-diastolic diameter, gender, ischemic cardiomyomyia, atrial fibrillation, and epicardial left ventricular electrode [139]. Another retrospective study of 2191 CRT patients evaluated the effect of gender differences and follow-up time on the predictive effect of machine learning models. The investigators found that the working AUC of random forest models for predicting all-cause death at 1 and 3 years was 0.728 (95% CI: 0.645–0.802) and 0.732 (95% CI: 0.681–0.784), respectively. Serum sodium level, hemoglobin concentration, age, heart failure etiology, NYHA classification, LVEF, and QRS morphology were the most important predictors of all-cause mortality risk. The order of importance of these features was influenced by gender differences and differed at 1 and 3 years of follow-up [140]. At present, the limitations of these algorithms are due to the particularity of the enrolled population, and it is unclear whether these algorithms are applicable to all CRT patients. In addition, the above results indicate that the risk prediction effect of the random forest model will be affected by the type and number of included variables. To corroborate, its prediction effect will also be affected by the extension of follow-up time. Therefore, these results need to be validated in other study populations and discussed at different follow-up times. If applicable to the clinic, these results will help physicians make optimal clinical decisions before CRT implantation.

#### 3.7.2.2 AI-ECG in Differential Diagnosis of Implantable Cardioverter Defibrillators

For implantable cardioverter-defibrillators (ICDs), it is important to distinguish between supraventricular tachycardia (SVT) and ventricular tachycardia (VT). This is because an inappropriate shock can cause great pain to the patient and may induce a life-threatening tachyarrhythmia. The MA-DIT II study showed that among 719 ICD patients, 11.5% of them had inappropriate shocks, and improper shocks accounted for the majority (31.2%) of the total number of shocks [141]. Based on the support vector calculation method, French scholars constructed a new two-dimensional intracavity graph (EGM) tracing method for single-cavity ICD to identify SVT and VT. The accuracy and sensitivity of the algorithm were 98.8% and 91.3%, respectively [142]. Mahajan et al. conducted a study employing 776 instances of arrhythmia events to develop an algorithmic model. They further validated this model with 131 cases involving incidents of electric shock in double-cavity ICDs. The study's findings revealed that no significant disparity existed between the accuracy of electrophysiological experts and the algorithm in distinguishing between VT/VF and non-VT/VF cases, even when referencing atrial electrogram (EGM) data (94% vs. 95%, $P = 0.87$). Similarly, no statistically significant distinction was observed between the accuracy of electrophysiologists and the algorithm in identifying VT/VF or non-VT/VF cases in scenarios where atrial EGM reference was absent (90% vs. 91%, $P = 0.91$) [143]. Hence, even in the absence of atrial EGM information, the machine learning algorithm maintained its noteworthy capability for accurate recognition.

#### 3.7.2.3 AI's Application in Selecting Candidates for ICD Placement

In the context of individuals at elevated risk of sudden cardiac death, ICDs play a pivotal role by promptly detecting and delivering defibrillation shocks to restore normal heart rhythm following severe ventricular arrhythmias. The accurate identification of the high-risk segment susceptible to sudden cardiac death, along with the prevention of such events through ICD implantation, holds significant clinical importance. While the current approach to primary prevention of sudden cardiac death largely revolves around reduced LVEF, this method exhibits limited predictive efficacy [144] and restricts understanding of ventricular arrhythmia pathogenesis. Consequently, researchers have turned to AI-driven algorithms, which leverage intricate interconnections among various risk factors to effectively identify high-risk populations. Wu et al. employed baseline and follow-up data from 382 patients with cardiomyopathy to develop a random forest model for predicting appropriate ICD interventions. This model was then compared with the Seattle Heart Failure Model score, leading to the discovery that the random forest model exhibited the highest predictive accuracy, boasting a median area under the curve (AUC) of 0.88 (95% CI: 0.75–0.96). Notably, the most influential predictors included not only heart failure-related hospitalizations but also factors like left ventricular scarring, left ventricular volume, left atrial volume, left atrial function, and interleukin-6 levels. These findings offer a novel foundation for effectively identifying individuals at heightened risk of sudden cardiac death.

#### 3.7.2.4 AI's Application in Selecting Candidates for Pacemaker Implantation Post-TAVR

In the context of patients experiencing atrioventricular block subsequent to transcatheter aortic valve replacement (TAVR), the necessity for permanent pacemaker implantation (PPI) arises. Clinicians are tasked with stratifying the risk for such patients before surgical intervention. However, the establishment of precise risk prediction methodologies remains elusive. Tsushima et al. conducted a retrospective analysis encompassing 888 patients who underwent TAVR between March 2011 and October 2018. Among them, 184 necessitated cardiac implantable electronic device treatment following TAVR. The researchers meticulously constructed and juxtaposed various algorithms, including decision tree, random forest, naive Bayes, multi-layer perceptron, k-nearest neighbor, local weight learning, and logistic regression. The findings underscored that logistic regression and naive Bayes exhibited the most robust predictive efficacy [145]. Similarly, Truong et al. undertook a continuous analysis involving 557 patients subjected to TAVR for severe aortic stenosis. The patient cohort, with a median age of 80 years, comprised 52% men, and 95 individuals necessitated PPI post-surgery. Leveraging preoperative and postoperative clinical data from TAVR, the researchers devised both random forest and logistic regression models. Upon comparison, the predictive potency of the random forest model outperformed that of the logistic regression model (AUC: 0.81 vs. 0.69) [146].

#### 3.7.2.5 AI in Distinguishing His Bundle Pacing Sites

His bundle pacing (HBP) is a pacing technique that directly stimulates the His bundle and Purkinje fibers through pacing wires. Due to its physiological pacing characteristics, HBP can serve as an alternative to traditional ventricular pacing [147]. However, HBP offers three distinct pacing modes: selective HBP, non-selective HBP, and myocardium-only capture. Accurately distinguishing between these modes is crucial for surgeons to identify the optimal electrode implantation site, albeit a challenging task. Arnold et al. conducted an analysis of 1297 electrocardiograms (ECGs) from 59 patients to develop a neural network model capable of automatically discerning these three pacing modes. The outcomes demonstrated that the neural network algorithm achieved accuracies of 67% for selective HBP, 71% for non-selective HBP, and 84% for myocardium-only capture [148]. Consequently, AI-powered automated ECG analysis holds the potential to assist HBP, mitigating complications arising from inappropriate pacing.

#### 3.7.2.6 AI for Enhanced Remote Follow-Up Optimization

AI algorithms offer the potential for optimizing remote follow-up procedures. Remote monitoring of patients with cardiac implantable electronic devices (CIEDs) contributes to the early detection of arrhythmias and technical device issues, thereby enhancing patient follow-up and prognosis. Despite these benefits, the integration of CIED remote follow-up into clinical practice has been hindered by factors such as medical costs and reimbursement challenges. Additionally, the extensive monitoring and alarm management associated with remote follow-up can impose a considerable time burden on physicians and experienced administrators. Rosier [149], a French researcher, attempted to develop an AI-driven atrial fibrillation risk classification alarm system. By extracting medical records and creating a model, the study categorized atrial fibrillation risk into four grades: low, medium, high, and extremely high. The researchers analyzed program-controlled records from 60 patients with implanted pacemakers and combined them with the CHA2DS2-VASc score and atrial fibrillation duration for manual risk grading. The study's outcomes showcased the smart model's capability to accurately classify 98% of pacemaker alerts, resulting in an 84% reduction in manual workload while ensuring patient safety. As the clinical dataset expands, the application of machine learning algorithms is anticipated to further enhance diagnostic and treatment accuracy within the realm of cardiac electrophysiology and pacing.

### 3.7.3 Summary

The integration of machine learning tools with clinical data offers the potential to create standardized predictive models, aiding experts in cardiac electrophysiology and pacing to formulate patient-specific guidelines. This approach, when compared to traditional research methods, serves as an extension of statistical understanding, utilizing AI to enhance rather than replace medical professionals in clinical decision-making. It is crucial for doctors to comprehend how to effectively utilize AI to test hypotheses, conduct comprehensive big data analyses, and optimize its application within clinical settings. Currently, these models require validation across diverse clinical datasets, with ongoing expansion of training datasets aimed at refining the accuracy of model predictions, diagnoses, classifications, and more.

## 3.8 Identification of Hypertension and Continuous Blood Pressure Monitoring

Bin Zhou and Min Tang

Cardiovascular disease stands as the primary global cause of mortality, responsible for approximately 17.9 million deaths each year, constituting 31% of total worldwide fatalities [150]. High blood pressure, a significant risk factor for cardiovascular ailments, necessitates early detection. Alas, hypertension's prevalence continues to increase due to aging demographics, inadequate awareness, and limited cure rates [151, 152]. Timely and dependable blood pressure measurement is imperative for reducing the incidence of hypertension and its associated cardiovascular complications. Monitoring crucial heart health indicators, including blood pressure and heart rate, has proven pivotal for the prevention and diagnosis of cardiovascular diseases [153, 154]. Effectively identifying specific conditions, such as "hidden" and "white coat" hypertension, is essential. Both are profoundly linked to escalated cardiovascular risk [155]. The prevalence of concealed hypertension ranges from 8% to 20%, affecting up to 50% of treated hypertensive patients. The recommendation commonly centers on continuous or ambulatory blood pressure monitoring to accurately identify these individuals [153]. However, conventional ambulatory blood pressure monitoring devices typically employ oscillatory techniques that entail repeated arm inflations. The discomfort and potential pain associated with these devices, particularly during sleep, have constrained their application in routine healthcare. Consequently, there is a growing demand for solutions that offer uninterrupted and continuous blood pressure monitoring [156].

ECG, as a widely employed clinical tool for assessing heart function, offers the advantages of being non-invasive and cost-effective. In clinical settings, electrophysiologists, possessing extensive expertise, often interpret ECG signals. However, this process is time-intensive and heavily reliant on individual subjectivity. In the contemporary landscape of healthcare technology, the trend is shifting toward quantifying and automating the analysis of ECG signals to assist clinicians in evaluating patient risk. Recent years have witnessed the escalating role of AI in healthcare, driven by the exponential growth of diverse electronic health data types [157]. Furthermore, advancements in hardware technology over the past decade, exemplified by robust computing platforms like cloud computing, high-performance computing, graphics processing units, and efficient modern software technologies, have facilitated the emergence of new technologies across various domains. Notably, deep learning, a subfield of AI, has gained significant traction [158]. Rooted in data analysis and pattern recognition, these technologies have achieved remarkable success in domains such as speech recognition [158] and image analysis [159].

Numerous studies have proposed the integration of AI for hypertension identification and blood pressure monitoring, utilizing ECG signals alone or in conjunction with other signals such as photoplethysmography (PPG). This section systematically explores prevalent AI methodologies and relevant research pertaining to ECG-based recognition and monitoring of blood pressure.

### 3.8.1 Traditional Machine Learning and Deep Learning in AI

AI involves the emulation of human cognitive processes using machines. AI machines are capable of thinking and performing tasks in a manner similar to humans, encompassing a wide array of functions. Machine learning (ML) is a method through which machines autonomously learn and enhance their performance based on experience, devoid of explicit human programming to define rules and logic. On the other hand, deep learning (DL) is a subset of ML characterized by its utilization of multiple layers of non-linear processing units for the extraction and transformation of features. Each consecutive layer employs the output from the preceding layer as its input.

In traditional machine learning, feature extraction is manually performed, while training is conducted using the extracted features. Various traditional machine learning algorithms are utilized, including the following: (1) Decision Tree (DT): A supervised model predicting targets based on a tree-like structure composed of nodes and branches. When predicting a continuous target variable, it is known as decision tree regression (DTR). (2) K-Nearest Neighbor (KNN): Classifies features based on the most prevalent groups among k-nearest neighbors. (3) Linear Discriminant Analysis (LDA): Predicts outcomes by estimating the probability of new data belonging to each category, with the highest probability determining the final output. (4) Linear Regression (LR): A simple regression algorithm with interpretability and minimal demand for training samples, making it fast and efficient for training. However, it may not be suitable for strong non-linear relationships between features and targets. (5) Support Vector Regression (SVR): Minimizes error within boundary lines using hyperplanes to segregate the dataset. (6) Random Forest (RF): Generates predictions by combining outcomes from multiple weak learners, such as decision trees, in parallel. To reduce bias and prediction variance, each tree is trained on a random subset of the training data, and the average of predictions serves as the final result. (7) Adaptive Boosting (AdaBoost): An iterative algorithm training different classifiers (weak classifiers) on the same dataset, and then assembling them to create a stronger final classifier (strong classifier). AdaBoost models are less prone to overfitting and require fewer training samples compared to more complex models.

In contrast to traditional machine learning techniques that rely on manually engineered features, artificial neural networks within the field of deep learning possess the ability to automatically extract relevant features from input data. However, this automated feature extraction capability is limited by reduced interpretability. Deep learning encompasses architectures with multiple layers, and among them, fully connected neural networks (FNN) and convolutional neural networks (CNNs) are particularly popular [158]. Recurrent neural networks (RNNs), a subset of neural networks, excel at capturing temporal characteristics present in signals, making them suitable for processing time series data like electrocardiograms (ECG). This capacity led to the proposal of a model that combines convolutional layers with long short-term memory (LSTM) layers, an architecture within RNNs for ECG diagnosis [160]. This fusion allows for effective processing of ECG time series data, demonstrating the adaptability and power of deep learning in medical applications.

Different machine learning approaches come with their own set of advantages and disadvantages. In the context of ECG classification, the efficacy of traditional machine learning is heavily reliant on the capacity to represent extracted ECG features. Since the predictive significance of each extracted feature varies, the results derived from traditional machine learning models are open to clinical interpretation [161]. On the contrary, deep learning operates by utilizing data to autonomously learn optimal features and parameters for specific tasks. However, these learned features and parameters often lack direct interpretability. The inability to establish explanations for the functional dependencies between inputs and outputs is known as the "black box" phenomenon. While deep learning can yield exceptional performance, the trade-off is the reduced ability to extract meaningful insights from the model's inner workings.

### 3.8.2 Identification of Hypertension and Blood Pressure Monitoring Using Single ECG Signals

Desmond et al. [162] developed an intelligent computing tool designed to use ECG signals for the detection of hypertension and possibly hidden hypertension. In this study, ECG signals were first collected from both normal and hypertensive people. After signal processing, non-linear features were extracted from five inherent modal functions. The T-test was then used to select a set of highly distinguishable features. Finally, the feature set was fed into three different machine learning algorithms (DT, KNN, and LDA). After calculation, the accuracy of KNN was found to be the highest, reaching a value of 97.70%. The developed tools were evaluated by a tenfold cross-validation technique. The study showed that a tool developed with a single ECG signal alone could enable the classification of hypertension from normal ECG signals.

Miao et al. [163] proposed a method for continuous blood pressure monitoring based on a single-channel ECG signal. This approach incorporates a deep learning network that combines residual network (ResNet) and long short-term memory (LSTM) architectures. Initially, the original ECG signal underwent noise filtering, signal segmentation, and normalization. The features learned from the ECG signals using ResNet were input into a bidirectional LSTM network. The LSTM's output features were then utilized by a two-layer fully connected network for blood pressure prediction. To enhance prediction accuracy, the model was calibrated using participants' baseline blood pressure. The model was trained on an intensive care unit dataset and validated on an independent test set. Results indicated that the proposed method achieved an estimated error of (0.07 ± 7.77 mmHg) for mean arterial pressure (MAP) and (0.01 ± 6.29 mmHg) for diastolic blood pressure (DBP), which satisfies the medical instrument standard (AAMI). When compared to traditional machine learning, deep learning models outperformed by identifying depth features with numerous parameters. The combination model of ResNet and LSTM proved more efficient in identifying depth features compared to using architecture individually. This approach offers accurate, reliable, and implementable continuous blood pressure monitoring through a single-channel ECG signal. It paves the way for convenient and precise blood pressure measurement using wearable devices in the future.

### 3.8.3 Combining ECG Signals and Other Signals to Identify Hypertension and Monitor Blood Pressure

In non-invasive blood pressure monitoring, PPG is the most common physiological signal used in the combined ECG. A number of studies have proposed non-invasive methods for blood pressure monitoring based on both ECG and PPG channels. Pulse conduction time (PTT) is the most widely used parameter for non-invasive BP monitoring. PTT refers to the time it takes for a pulse wave to travel between two locations in the cardiovascular system, which can be calculated based on two pulse signals generated by the cardiovascular system, such as ECG and PPG. Based on PTT, a multi-parameter model can be constructed from various parameters extracted from ECG and PPG signals. Zhang et al. [164] proposed a method to estimate blood pressure using multiple physiological parameters, taking into account the regulation of the sympathetic nervous system on vascular activity. The parameters used in this model include heart rate variability (HRV), PTT, and pulse wave morphological features extracted from ECG/PPG signals. Four classical machine learning algorithms were used in this study, including LR, SVR, RF, and AdaBoost. A mixed dataset of 3337 subjects from two databases was evaluated using these four classical machine learning algorithms to verify the ability to migrate across databases. In addition, separate calibration procedures were employed to further improve the accuracy of the method. The results show that the AdaBoost and RF algorithms perform equally and better than the other two algorithms. The mean absolute error (MAE) and root mean square error (RMSE) of the AdaBoost algorithm are 10.03 mmHg and 14.55 mmHg of systolic blood pressure (SBP) and 5.42 mmHg and 8.19 mmHg of diastolic blood pressure (DBP), respectively. When calibrated separately, MAE and standard deviation are 0.16 ± 7.96 mmHg for SBP and 0.13 ± 4.5 mmHg for DBP, respectively, meeting the AAMI standard. In addition, these models were used to test individual databases to evaluate their performance on different data sources. The Adaboost algorithm performed well overall in the critical care unit multi-parameter intelligent monitoring database (MIMIC), with MAE between the predicted and true values of 6.6 mmHg and 3.12 mmHg for SBP and DBP, respectively. The method proposed by the institute considers the regulation of blood vessels and the heart by the autonomic nervous system, which is promising for improving the accuracy of continuous and interference-free blood pressure estimation.

Liu et al. [165] used ECG and PPG signals to construct a multi-parameter fusion-based method for continuous blood pressure measurement in patients with arrhythmia. The study extracted 15 features from ECG and PPG signals and used four machine learning algorithms, including DTR, SVR, Adaboost, and RF. The performance of each model was evaluated based on the mean and standard deviation of RSME. Compared with the DTR (7.68 ± 3.91 mmHg) and SVR (7.63 ± 4.1 mmHg) models, the RF model performed better in the estimation of SBP (5.87 ± 3.13 mmHg). However, although the RSME estimated by SBP for the RFR model was also smaller than the RSME (6.24 ± 3.22 mmHg) for Adaboost, the difference was not significant. In addition, the RSME of the RF model in the DBP estimate was calculated at 3.52 ± 1.38 mmHg, which is comparable to the values using the SVR (3.88 ± 1.35 mmHg) and Adaboost (3.62 ± 1.28 mmHg) models. However, it was significantly smaller than the DTR model (4.44 ± 1.56 mmHg). Therefore, the RF-based RSME in the BP estimate exhibited better performance (i.e., lower RSME) and faster training capability compared to the Adaboost model; hence, it was selected as the best blood pressure estimation algorithm. The proposed approach was further evaluated against the AAMI criteria and the British Hypertension Society (BHS) criteria. Overall, the mean and standard deviation of the difference between the SBP and DBP estimates and the actual values were 0.04 ± 6.11 mmHg and 0.11 ± 3.62 mmHg, respectively. This suggests that the methods used for the

SBP and DBP estimates satisfy the AAMI criteria for patients with arrhythmia in the current situation. The SBP and DBP estimates of the proposed method meet Class A criteria based on the BHS criteria. This study suggests that a multi-parameter model based on ECG and PPG using machine learning algorithms (RF) can effectively monitor blood pressure in the case of arrhythmia.

Li et al. [166] proposed a deep learning model based on ECG and PPG for real-time estimation of SBP and DBP. The data for this model came from the Critical Care database (MIMIC II). The model contains a bidirectional LSTM at the first layer, followed by an N-layer LSTM. The remaining connections are made for each LSTM layer by inputting seven parameters based on the ECG and PPG waveform characteristics. At the same time, the performance of the model was compared with three traditional machine learning models and another existing deep learning model. The study shows that the model was superior to existing methods and contained the potential to assist in future clinical practice.

### 3.8.4 Current Problems and Prospects

At present, there are many studies using AI to identify hypertension and continuously monitor blood pressure based on ECG, with or without PPG signal. The basic research process is shown in Fig. 3.1. Most of the studies have shown the feasibility of the proposed models, but there is currently no recognized model for clinical practice. Possible problems include the following: (1) Diseases, drugs, individual differences, and other factors that may have affected the change in blood pressure. Therefore, the baseline characteristics of each patient should be considered during the development of the blood pressure model, and changes in medication should be taken into account. (2) The signals and reference blood pressure values collected in the clinical setting may have some noise characteristics, hence influencing the stability of the model. Therefore, data preprocessing procedures should be performed prior to model development to reduce noise and remove signals of poor quality. (3) Given the variation in hemodynamic responses to changes in blood pressure between individuals, most studies had adopted individualized model modeling, which limits the external clinical applicability of the proposed models. (4) With the exception of a few studies using publicly available databases, most studies have limited sample sizes, making it difficult to develop population models. In the future, large clinical multicenter studies may be needed to propose models with wider applicability.

Despite the aforementioned problems, with the continuous development of AI, there will be more opportunities for using wearable devices in the healthcare field. The direction of non-invasive blood pressure monitoring based on simple and easily accessible ECG signals is promising. At the same time, studies using AI to extract ECG signals have been used for atrial fibrillation recognition, hypertrophic cardiomyopathy recognition, age/gender recognition, left atrial enlargement recognition, etc. If the AI algorithm for hypertension recognition and blood pressure monitoring can be combined with the above scenarios, an application system for the whole cardiovascular scene can be created to benefit more patients.

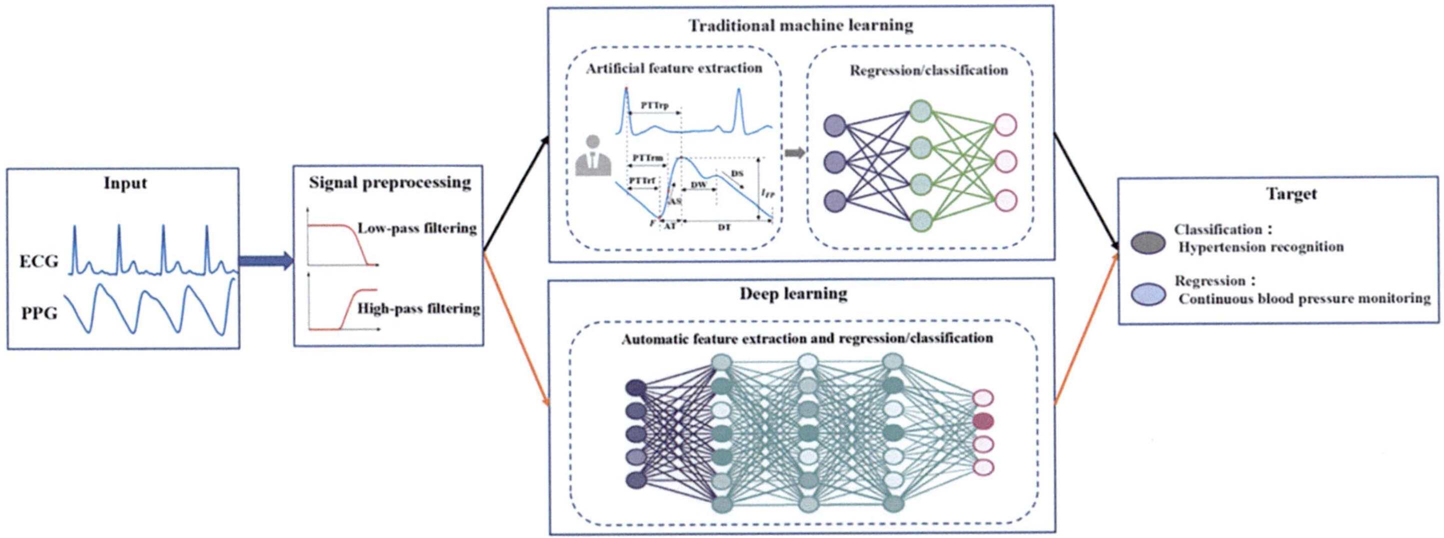


**Fig. 3.1** The routine research process of using AI to identify hypertension and continuously monitor blood pressure based on ECG with or without pulse wave. *ECG* electrocardiograph, *PPG* photoplethysmography, *PTT* pulse transit time, *AT* ascending time, *DT* descending time, *AS* ascending slope, *DS* descending slope, *IFP* PPG peak-foot point intensity difference, *DW* large artery stiffness index

## 3.9 Atrial Fibrillation

Hui-Min Chu and Bin-Hao Wang

Atrial fibrillation (AF) is the most common arrhythmia disease, which can increase the risk of stroke, heart failure, and death [167]. There are still some challenges in its early identification, diagnosis, and treatment. Traditional screening methods have great limitations and greatly underestimate the prevalence of AF. Despite the continuous improvement of monitoring methods, the prevalence of AF continues to rise. Subsequently, a large amount of resources and time is dedicated to processing patients' clinical data, medication information, and other information. Based on these data, doctors can formulate individualized treatment plans for patients, but there are great challenges in using traditional statistical tools to process big data. AI algorithms can overcome some of these existing limitations and, in recent years, have begun to emerge in the field of AF diagnosis and treatment.

### 3.9.1 Common Technologies

As a branch of computer science, AI includes machine learning, deep learning, etc. Machine learning is produced by the interaction of statistics and computer science. Its research enables computers to rely on experience to learn and continuously optimize their own capabilities to achieve the purpose of simulating human learning. The general process is divided into data preprocessing, feature selection, data classification, simulation training, and optimization. Machine learning techniques are mainly divided into three types: supervised learning, unsupervised learning, and reinforcement learning. (1) Supervised learning: Learn or suggest a model from training data and infer new instances in turn. The task of supervised learning is to rely on correctly labeled training data to obtain an output for any possible input value. The output result may be a prediction or classification. For example, data training is performed on the ECG of a group of patients diagnosed with AF, and the final model can be used to judge whether there is AF in the newly imported ECG. (2) Unsupervised learning: No need to predict the results; the main purpose is to discover the basic results and relationships between different variables in the data. In this approach, the input data is unlabeled, the output data is unknown, and the system relies on the basis of the data to look for specific patterns. Cluster analysis is a commonly used algorithm for unsupervised learning that can classify research objects according to certain standards, and each category has its corresponding characteristics. For example, a group of patients with AF is stratified for stroke risk according to clinical data. (3) Reinforcement learning is a machine learning paradigm that involves learning by interacting with an environment through a cyclical process of experimentation. This framework consists of a defined environment and an agent that operates within it in real time. When the agent takes an action within the environment, the environment responds by altering its state. Simultaneously, the environment generates a reinforcement signal that provides feedback to the agent.

The agent utilizes this reinforcement signal in conjunction with the current state of the environment to make informed decisions, thereby selecting the subsequent action to take.

Deep learning is a new research field in machine learning, aiming to build a neural network similar to the human brain, including neural network (NN), CNN, etc. (1) NN: Simulate the connection mode between neurons in the human brain to form a blood transfusion model that combines many signal calculation units. NN is composed of a large number of processing units arranged in a multi-layer structure, with the layers connecting to each other through certain weights, and the input data is processed to produce corresponding results. (2) CNN: It is the most widely used type of deep learning model. It imitates the biological visual perception mechanism, holding great advantages in image and audio data feature extraction through multiple convolution calculations.

### 3.9.2 Application of AI in the Diagnosis of AF

The traditional diagnostic methods of AF mainly include cardiac examination and ECG. A 12-lead ECG is the gold standard for diagnosing AF. The diagnosis is made based on the RR interval and P wave of the ECG. However, due to the sharp increase in the number of patients, doctors sometimes cannot make an accurate diagnosis for a large number of ECGs. In addition, some patients with AF are paroxysmal; thus, ordinary 12-lead ECG or 24-h dynamic ECG may not be able to record the onset of AF, resulting in a missed diagnosis. Implantable ECG event recorders can extend the monitoring time to 3 years; however, it is expensive and is an invasive operation, which imposes a burden on patients and clinical work. If patients with AF cannot be diagnosed in time, they may not receive timely treatments such as anticoagulants, which could lead to thromboembolic events in severe cases. Therefore, we urgently need a non-invasive, cheap, and simple monitoring method.

Machine learning can improve the accuracy of feature extraction and identify the cardiac rhythm changes on the 12-lead or single-lead ECG. Hannun et al. [168] imported 91,232 single-lead ECG records into a CNN to create a model for distinguishing 12 different heart rhythms (including AF) and found that the AUC of the model predicting heart rhythm was as high as 0.91. The model was then integrated into NN software and coded into the hardware of wearable devices to collect signals through photoplethysmography and conduct cardiac rhythm analysis [169–171]. Apple Inc. of the United States launched a clinical study on the monitoring of AF with wearable devices. The study included 419,297 participants. All subjects identified as having AF received ECG examinations, and 34% of them were clinically diagnosed as having AF, with a positive predictive value of 0.84 [170]. In addition, the results of a domestic study on the use of smart bracelets to screen for AF (HUAWEI Heart Study) have also been published. Among 187,912 individuals using smart bracelets, 424 patients with "suspected AF" were screened out, and 262 of them received medical treatment. A total of 227 cases of AF were diagnosed through institutional inspection, with a positive predictive value of 91.6% [169]. In addition, ECG recording via wearable devices is now possible. Kardiaband paired with an Apple Watch can record a single-lead ECG. A study of 24 patients with paroxysmal AF showed that the sensitivity of the device to identify AF episodes ≥1 h was 97.5% [172]. The above studies confirmed the feasibility of wearable devices for AF monitoring.

In addition, before the occurrence of AF, there may be changes in the structure of the atrium, such as myocardial hypertrophy and fibrosis. These may cause subtle electrical changes in the heart, which can be reflected on the ECG. Studies suggest that AI may be able to identify AF from a normal rhythm ECG. In a study published in *The Lancet*, researchers developed an AI model that can detect signs of AF from ECGs of patients in sinus rhythm. The researchers used 650,000 ECGs (standard 12-lead, 10 s) from 181,000 patients and divided them into two groups according to whether they had AF. Then, the NN was used to identify the subtle changes of ECG under sinus rhythm by constructing NN. ECG data is divided into three groups, namely, training (70%), internal validation (10%), and test (20%) data. It was finally found that the accuracy of the AI model in identifying AF was as high as 83% [10]. This study suggests that AI applied to ECG can detect AF. Even if AF does not occur when ECG is recorded, the AI model can identify subtle changes and predict potential patients with AF.

The above research results suggest that with the continuous development of AI, it may be possible to identify high-risk patients with AF by analyzing sinus rhythm ECG at an early stage. For these patients, it is recommended to wear wearable devices and seek medical treatment in a timely manner after abnormalities are found.

### 3.9.3 Application of AI in AF Ablation

It is very necessary to evaluate the condition of the left atrium and related anatomy by imaging examination before AF ablation. Manual processing of imaging data will consume a lot of time and may cause certain errors [173, 174]; however, AI technology can well overcome this limitation [175]. Most centers in China will perform left atrium CT to clarify the anatomy of the pulmonary veins before surgery. Chen et al. used deep CNN to build a model that automatically recognizes CT images and reconstructs the three-dimensional anatomical structure of the left atrium. The study found that the model is accurate in identifying the structure of the left atrium in CT images. The accuracy was 99%, the sensitivity was 99.3%, and the specificity was 98.7% [176]. In recent years, the application of cardiac magnetic resonance technology in patients with AF has gradually increased. This includes quantitative analysis of data, three-dimensional reconstruction, and the combination of delayed gadolinium. Enhanced sequences can also be used to assess the degree of left atrial fibrosis and guide ablation strategies for AF. Bai et al. used a CNN image segmentation algorithm to process cardiac MRI image sequences of 5008 patients. Compared with manual processing, CNN can not only significantly reduce processing time but also greatly improve accuracy [173]. In addition, AI also has a greater advantage in the identification of left atrial scar regions. Valinoti et al. used deep learning technology to automatically integrate left atrium segmentation and left atrial scar area identification. The data imported was processed through a three-dimensional guidance system, which is conducive to shortening the operation time and performing individualized ablation [177]. The above studies show that the application of AI in imaging examinations before AF ablation has its unique advantages. Although the above techniques are promising, they still need to be validated in patients with different anatomical structures. Also, standard intervals for relevant parameters should be explored.

Electrophysiological matrix mapping of the left atrium is required in AF ablation, and the interpretation of the results is highly subjective, resulting in differences among different operators and differences in ablation procedures. In recent years, AI has been gradually applied to the analysis of mapping results, and machine learning is used to automatically analyze the time-space activation model of the left atrium to guide ablation. A study trained a supervised learning CNN to classify data from 35 patients with persistent AF to identify effective ablation sites for terminating AF. The study found that the prediction accuracy of the model reached 95% [178]. Previous studies have shown that the presence of external pulmonary vein triggers is an important predictor of AF recurrence after ablation, and ablation of these triggers can improve the success rate of surgery. Liu et al. included 358 patients with paroxysmal AF who had undergone catheter ablation and had no recurrence 1 year after surgery. They divided the patients into two groups according to whether there were external trigger lesions in the pulmonary veins. They applied deep learning to the CT images of the pulmonary veins before ablation. Analyzed and predicted the existence of trigger foci outside the pulmonary veins, it was found that the prediction accuracy of the model was 82.4 ± 2.0%, the sensitivity was 64.3 ± 5.4%, and the specificity was 88.4 ± 1.9% [179].

### 3.9.4 Application of AI in Individualized Treatment of AF

In recent years, the AF guidelines issued by major associations all emphasize individualized comprehensive management, including symptom management, drug therapy (control of ventricular rate, antiarrhythmic, and anticoagulant drugs), device therapy (left atrial appendage occlusion and pacing treatment), etc. [180, 181]. In the past, patients were usually classified according to the type of AF, but it could not fully reflect the individual differences among patients. At present, there has been some exploration of using unsupervised AI technology in the management of AF, which can be classified and individualized according to patient data. One study included about 10,000 patients, who were divided into four categories according to baseline data: (1) AF patients with fewer risk factors and comorbid diseases; (2) AF patients who were young and/or had behavioral disorders; (3) AF patients with fast-slow syndrome and symptoms requiring device implantation; and (4) AF patients with coronary artery disease, acute myocardial infarction, and/or atherosclerosis. It was found that compared with patients in the first category, the risk of major cardiovascular events, nervous system events, and major bleeding events was higher in the remaining three groups, which should attract the attention of clinicians [182].

AI can not only play a role in patient risk assessment and group management but also help supervise patients to standardize their medication. In the past 10 years, new oral anticoagulant drugs have become more and more widely used, and they tend to replace warfarin. Some people with AF (end-stage renal disease, valvular AF, etc.) can only take warfarin for anticoagulation, but the application of warfarin still has certain challenges. Different individuals have different starting doses of warfarin, and machine learning algorithms can provide appropriate warfarin doses for different individuals based on demographic, clinical, and pharmaceutical data [183, 184]. In addition, patients' compliance with anticoagulant drugs is poor, and a considerable number of patients stop taking the drugs after a period of time. With the application of new oral anticoagulant drugs in clinical practice, medication compliance has improved to some extent, but the range is not large [185].

Labovitz et al. combined smartphones with AI technology to intervene in patients taking medicine. Through the above-mentioned measures, patients were video-monitored to confirm taking medicine. The results found that the compliance of patients in the intervention group was as high as 100% after taking medicine, while only 50% of patients took the medicine through the traditional method [186]. Patients with AF often use antiarrhythmic drugs and require close monitoring of cardiac parameters, subsequently adjusting drug treatment accordingly. These factors include QT interval, suitability for QT interval prolonging drugs, renal function, etc. This is intended to prevent arrhythmia adverse reactions such as abnormalities; however, the QT interval alone cannot accurately reflect the patient's blood drug concentration. A study used ECG data to predict the blood concentration of dofetilide by establishing a deep learning model and found a good correlation with the real blood concentration [187]. Levy et al. used a machine learning model to obtain the dosage of dofetilide for each patient, and the accuracy of the recommended dosage was 96.1% [188].

### 3.9.5 Current Challenges

The huge amount of data makes the clinical decisions given by the AI model seem more convincing, but the current limitations of AI in clinical applications are also very prominent. First, medical ethics issues must be acknowledged. A large amount of data includes clinical data of patients, and some information may involve patient privacy. Therefore, it is best to obtain informed consent from patients before using their data, but due to the large sample size, it will undoubtedly increase the huge workload. Second, data quality issues may raise concerns for the model design. Massive database extraction is a key feature of AI models, and accurate data collection is crucial. If there are varying degrees of quality problems in the collected data, the accuracy of the direct use of the AI model will naturally be lowered, making the model unable to extract large-scale cohort data. For example, there may be some differences in the ECG data, varying positions of the ECG lead placed by different inspectors, and the measurement standard of the ECG waveform quality. Therefore, standardization during data collection is crucial. Third, the "black box" phenomenon of machine learning is a great limitation of AI usage. After inputting data, although the model shows an output prediction result, we don't know how the machine has processed this outcome. Moreover, at present, AI algorithms are generally carried out by information technology personnel, and few clinicians are involved; hence, the conclusions drawn may lack clinical practical value. In medicine, where evidence-based evidence is critical, clinical recommendations derived from machine learning alone may be difficult for clinicians to adopt. Fourth, the issue of generalization of results. At present, the clinical application of AI is still in its infancy. Many algorithms are only based on one database for research, and the breadth of the included population may be limited. In addition, there may be multiple algorithms for predicting the same disease. Whether it is suitable for different populations and whether it can be integrated is still unknown, which largely limits the promotion of the results to the whole population.

### 3.9.6 Summary and Outlook

In the field of cardiac electrophysiology, AI has been widely used in recent years, especially in the diagnosis and treatment of AF. With the continuous advancement of AI monitoring and diagnostic technology, a variety of wearable devices have entered our lives for the management of AF rhythm and heart rate. In addition, the application of AI in AF ablation has begun to be explored. For the processing of preoperative imaging examination data, AI has its unique advantages, which can help evaluate the degree of atrial fibrosis and automatically complete intraluminal matrix mapping. It is believed that with the continuous progress and innovation of AI technology, breaking through current limitations, it will carry promising implications for improving the diagnosis and treatment of AF in the future.

## 3.10 Heart Valve Disease

Bing-Xin Xie and Tong Liu

### 3.10.1 Basic Overview of Heart Valves

Valvular heart disease (VHD) is a clinically common organic heart disease, often involving the destruction of the integrity of one or more heart valves. This results in valve stenosis, regurgitation, or a combination of the two, including the aortic valve, mitral valve, tricuspid valve, and pulmonary valve. Common etiologies include heredity, infection, immunity, senile degenerative changes, and functional changes. According to a large-scale population study in the United States, 11,911 people were screened by echocardiography. The results showed that after adjusting age, the incidence of heart valve disease was about 2.5%, of which aortic valve stenosis accounted for 0.4%, aortic valve regurgitation flow accounted for 0.5%, mitral stenosis accounted for 0.1%, and mitral regurgitation accounted for 1.7%. With the aging population, the incidence of senile degenerative valve disease and functional disease is increasing rapidly. The incidence of heart valve disease before the age of 65 is <2%, while the incidence rate between 65 and 75 is 8.5% and 13.2%, respectively. Rheumatic valvular heart disease remains an important cause of valvular heart disease in developing countries [189].

If heart disease is not detected and treated in time, once symptoms appear, especially when combined with cardiac insufficiency, it will drastically worsen the patient's prognosis. At present, the screening method that has been used clinically is echocardiography, but not all patients undergo echocardiography when they see a doctor, so there are certain difficulties in its early detection. With the rapid development of AI technology, it has been widely used in clinical diagnosis and treatment. The use of machine learning approaches can improve accuracy in disease prediction with high credibility, which has significantly improved the diagnostic efficiency of certain diseases.

AI can intelligently perceive the surrounding environment and imitate and demonstrate human cognitive behaviors, such as learning and problem solving. Machine learning is a field of AI. It can obtain large-scale predictions by designing mathematical models and training them. The dataset [190] has been widely studied in the medical field and is involved in the diagnosis and prognosis prediction of various diseases. AI machine learning has made some progress in the diagnosis of various cardiovascular diseases, including machine learning, such as the prediction of atrial fibrillation, heart valve disease, pulmonary hypertension, left ventricular diastolic dysfunction, and other diseases through ECG.

## 3.10.2 Research Progress of AI-ECG in the Prediction and Diagnosis of Valvular Disease

### 3.10.2.1 AI-ECG Identification of Aortic Valve Stenosis

Aortic stenosis (AS) usually has characteristic manifestations during systole, and many patients may not seek medical attention until symptoms appear. Only 62% of patients with asymptomatic aortic stenosis can find a heart murmur [191], and whether the heart murmur can be accurately assessed is also closely related to the doctor's auscultation skills. Therefore, it is difficult to perform early identification of aortic valve stenosis, which affects timely treatment.

In 2021, Cohen-Shelly and other researchers from the Department of Cardiology at the Mayo Clinic in the United States developed AI-ECG using CNN to identify patients with moderate to severe aortic stenosis through AI-ECG technology [192].

The team selected patients aged ≥18 years from 1989 to 2019 in the Mayo Clinic database. Selected patients had to undergo transthoracic echocardiography and standard 12-lead ECG examination within 180 days. A total of 9723 patients (3.7%)

were diagnosed with moderate to severe aortic stenosis by cardiac ultrasound. The AI algorithm was used to learn the ECGs (50%) of 129,788 patients, and 25,893 patients' ECGs (10%) were used for internal verification. The algorithm was finally tested on 102,926 patients (40%). In the validation set, AI-ECG flagged aortic stenosis (AUC: 0.85) in 3833 (3.7%) patients with a sensitivity, specificity, and accuracy of 78%, 74%, and 74%, respectively. As the patient's age increases, the sensitivity of the AI algorithm to identify aortic stenosis by ECG increased and the specificity decreased. At any age, the AI-ECG technique had higher specificity and lower sensitivity in female patients compared with male patients. When the research team added age and gender parameters to the model, the model's AUC for identifying patients with aortic stenosis among non-hypertensive patients increased to 0.90. The model also predicted the onset of aortic stenosis, and among patients using this AI-ECG to predict aortic stenosis, patients with false positives have a greater 15-year risk of developing moderate to severe aortic stenosis than those identified as true twice that of negative patients.

Evidence suggests that the AI-ECG algorithm can diagnose and predict aortic valve stenosis. With the continuous optimization of the machine learning algorithm, it will gradually be used in clinical practice from clinical research in the future, which will help doctors understand the clinical condition of patients. Compared with echocardiography, ECG is more convenient to operate and less costly. It is more suitable for population screening and helps to screen out key groups for further inspection. It can save medical resources and is conducive to the early detection and diagnosis of diseases.

#### 3.10.2.2 AI-ECG Identification of Mitral Regurgitation

Mitral regurgitation (MR), which refers to the regurgitation of blood from the left ventricle to the left atrium during systole, is the most common valvular disease in developed countries. The incidence of mitral regurgitation in the general population is 1.7%, but the incidence rate is about 10% among people over the age of 70 years [193, 194]. With the continuous progression of mitral regurgitation, it can lead to heart failure and seriously affect the quality of life of patients. Early screening and prediction are very important for the progression of mitral regurgitation and the prevention of adverse outcomes.

At present, the diagnosis of mitral valve regurgitation is mainly discovered by echocardiography after the patient has symptoms of discomfort, which is a relatively late intervention period. Patients often seek treatment for heart failure-related symptoms such as fatigue and exertional dyspnea. Not all patients have murmurs in the auscultation area of the mitral valve. Cardiac ultrasound is relatively expensive and takes a long time to check, so it is difficult to use as a means of disease screening, which also limits the early detection of mitral valve regurgitation. It was found that compared with echocardiography, ECG is simpler, less costly, and easier to operate and is more suitable for early screening of mitral regurgitation.

A study published in the *Journal of Electrocardiology* in 2020 used AI in the field of ECG for early diagnosis and prediction of mitral regurgitation [194]. This study was a multi-center retrospective cohort study involving two hospitals, a cardiovascular teaching hospital and a community general hospital. The study enrolled adults who underwent simultaneous ECG and echocardiography within 4 weeks. The patients enrolled in the cardiovascular teaching hospital from October 2016 to March 2019 were split and included in the algorithm derivation and internal validation datasets, respectively. The patients who underwent echocardiography follow-up after the first assessment were included in the internal validation dataset, and patients who did not undergo echocardiography during follow-up were included in the derived dataset for the derivation and development process of the AI algorithm. After the algorithm development was completed, the study used the teaching hospital's internal verification dataset to verify the algorithm, evaluate the accuracy of the AI algorithm, and use the community general hospital data (including data from March 2017 to March 2019) as external verification. A total of 56,670 ECGs of 24,202 patients were used for the derivation and development of the AI algorithm, 3174 ECGs of 3174 patients were used for internal verification, and 10,865 ECGs of 10,865 patients were used for external verification. The diagnosis was targeted for moderate to severe mitral regurgitation.

AI algorithm detected mitral regurgitation with a ROCAUC of 0.816 and 0.877 when internally and externally validated, respectively, by analysis of the patient's standard 12-lead ECG. Using the AI algorithm to analyze the patient's single-lead ECG, the ROCAUC for diagnosing mitral regurgitation was 0.758 and 0.850, respectively. Among the 3157 patients who had not yet been diagnosed with mitral valve regurgitation, it was found through 27 months of follow-up that the probability of mitral valve regurgitation in the high-risk group judged by the algorithm was higher than that of low-risk patients (13.9% vs. 2.6%, $P < 0.001$). The sensitive area diagram of the AI algorithm analyzed on the ECG shows that the algorithm mainly collects P wave and T wave data of patients with mitral regurgitation and QRS wave dispersion data of patients without mitral regurgitation.

This study takes the ECG data captured by the algorithm and analyzes the sensitive area map, visualizes it, increases the transparency of the AI algorithm, changes the shortcomings of the previous deep learning algorithm, and increases transparency. The AI algorithm is used to analyze the key areas of the ECG for diagnosis and prediction of mitral valve regurgitation in patients, which improves the detection rate of mitral valve regurgitation. Subsequently, this helps clinicians to identify high-risk patients early and carry out targeted treatment or early prevention. Ultimately, this may help improve the prognosis of patients and reduce the occurrence of related adverse outcomes.

### 3.10.3 Future Outlook

With the continuous development of AI technology, various new instruments and equipment are constantly updated and improved. AI will become increasingly prevalent in various fields of medical care, from heart rate monitoring bracelets to 3D model printing of the heart outside the body. At present, for the diagnosis of heart valve diseases, AI technology mainly focuses on the use of CT or MRI to scan the valve before valve replacement surgery. When combined with AI, physicians can accurately reconstruct the patient's valve and use 3D printing technology to generate a more fitting patient valve. Moreover, AI can predict the possibility of postoperative complications according to the condition of the valve, so that the surgeon can better understand the condition of the patient's valve before the operation and can prepare in advance for possible events during or after the operation.

ECG, as a simple, non-invasive, and low-cost cardiac examination method in grass-roots hospitals. Its function is no longer limited to the diagnosis of arrhythmia and myocardial ischemia. By combining with AI and machine learning algorithms, this approach can effectively diagnose and predict a variety of valve diseases. In the future, AI models will gradually cover the diagnosis and prediction of various heart diseases, assisting clinicians in the diagnosis and treatment process. Essentially, this can help to improve the quality of life and prognosis of patients.

## 3.11 Electrolyte Disturbance

Guan-Yu Mu and Kang-Yin Chen

Electrolyte levels in the blood are tightly regulated and are essential for maintaining normal physiological functions of cells. Many diseases can lead to electrolyte disturbances, and severe electrolyte disturbances may lead to fatal arrhythmias and sudden cardiac death. In patients with kidney or heart disease, even slight changes in electrolyte levels can lead to hospitalization and death. Therefore, the diagnosis and monitoring of electrolyte disturbances is very important. Currently, the gold standard for diagnosis is laboratory testing of electrolyte concentrations, but laboratory testing is invasive, costly, and requires specialized equipment and infrastructure. Therefore, routine assessment of electrolytes using laboratory tests may not be the best way to monitor health status and prevent fatal adverse events.

The balance of transmembrane electrolytes determines the state of cardiomyocyte membranes and affects cardiac function and ECG form. Previous studies have shown that electrolyte imbalances can alter ECG shape. Based on this, deep learning models may assess electrolyte status based on such subtle ECG changes.

### 3.11.1 Abnormal Blood Potassium

In clinical practice, hyperkalemia and hypokalemia are common causes of sudden cardiac death. Therefore, timely identification and rapid correction of abnormal potassium levels are crucial. Major ECG associated with hypokalemia changes include decreased T wave amplitude, ST segment depression, T wave inversion, PR interval prolongation, and increased QT correction interval (QTc). Typical ECG of hyperkalemia performance from high peak T wave and QT interval shortening progresses to PR interval prolongation and P wave disappears, then QRS. The wave group expands, eventually forming a sine wave pattern. Although these ECG morphological changes are common in patients with abnormal potassium levels, even experienced clinicians often overlook relevant details. Therefore, more advanced deep learning models have been developed to improve the diagnosis of electrolyte disorders.

As early as 2015, Dillon et al. [195] found that ECG repolarization-related ECG indicators (including T wave amplitude, slope, T/R amplitude ratio, etc.) can be used to detect changes in blood potassium levels in hemodialysis patients. Small changes in serum potassium levels within the normal range can cause quantifiable changes in the ECG signal. The study detects a minimum of 0.2 mmol/L changes in blood potassium levels. This suggests that non-invasive monitoring of serum potassium concentration based on ECG changes is feasible.

Later, in 2016, Attia ZI et al. [196] developed a single-lead ECG model for non-invasive monitoring of serum potassium. The study performed ECG recordings and blood tests on hemodialysis patients and then developed a personalized processed single-channel ECG regression to ensemble models for predicting serum potassium. The overall model can be based on T wave characteristics to predict serum potassium levels. The absolute error in potassium values was 10% of the measured value for the individual model and 12% for the ensemble model. This further proves that the single-lead signal processing ECG can be used to predict serum potassium values.

In 2019, the Galloway CD team [19] evaluated the deep learning model in CKD patient ECG detection of performance in hyperkalemia. The most important aspect of deep learning is its ability to extract features and use various types of data (such as images, 2D data, and waveforms) to develop algorithms. In this study, only 2 articles of ECG lead-lead, a deep learning model detected hyperkalaemic AUC in patients with kidney disease for 0.853–0.883. This study shows that AI Applied to ECG can screen for hyperkalemia.

By 2020, based on the above deep learning foundation, Lin et al. [197] developed a deep learning model, ECG12Net, based on ECG performance to evaluate blood potassium concentration. ECG12Net is an 82-layer CNN with sensitivities of 95.6% and 84.5% and specificities of 81.6% and 96.0% for the diagnosis of severe hypokalemia and hyperkalemia, respectively. The models were shown to perform significantly better than clinicians. These findings suggest that a deep learning model based on 12-lead ECG can help physicians identify severe potassium abnormalities in a timely manner, thereby potentially reducing cardiac events.

Recently, Kwon et al. [198] also developed a deep learning model for detecting electrolyte imbalance using ECG and validated its performance in a multicenter study. The results showed that the AUCs of 12-lead ambulatory ECG for detecting hyperkalemia and hypokalemia were 0.945 and 0.866, respectively. The AUC values for external validation were 0.873 and 0.857, respectively. At the same time, the model helps visualize important ECG regions for detecting electrolyte imbalances. ECG in patients with hyperkalemia showed QRS prolongation, QTc prolongation, T wave axis shift to the right, PR prolongation, and tachycardia. In conclusion, growing evidence suggests that DLM can be used to detect and monitor the daily ECG of abnormal potassium.

The above-mentioned deep learning model developed by Kwon et al. can not only be applied to the monitoring of abnormal blood potassium but can also be used to predict the disturbance of blood sodium and blood calcium balance [198]. The AUCs of the 12-lead ambulatory ECG for detecting hypernatremia, hyponatremia, hypercalcemia, and hypocalcemia were 0.944, 0.885, 0.905, and 0.901, respectively. The AUC values for external validation were 0.839, 0.856, 0.831, and 0.813. The AUC values for the 6-lead ECG for detecting hypernatremia, hyponatremia, hypercalcemia, and hypocalcemia were 0.833, 0.851, 0.813, and 0.812, respectively. The AUCs for hypernatremia, hyponatremia, hypercalcemia, and hypocalcemia detected by single-lead ECG were 0.806, 0.839, 0.634, and 0.798, respectively. Meanwhile, DLM outperformed logistic regression and random forest models for both internal and external validation datasets. In addition, DLM analysis detected significant ECG regions for each electrolyte imbalance: abnormalities in serum sodium correlated with heart rate, atrial fibrillation, PR interval, QRS interval, QT interval, QTc, and T wave axis. Calcium abnormalities are related to heart rate, atrial fibrillation, QRS interval, QT interval, QTc, R wave axis, and T wave axis. Thus, deep learning can be applied to the diagnosis and monitoring of a wider variety of electrolyte balance disorders.

In conclusion, new technologies and developments in AI are gradually being applied to ECG to diagnose electrolyte disturbances. This model will help doctors identify electrolyte disorders in time to reduce the occurrence of adverse outcomes. Ultimately, collaboration between doctors and AI can optimize the quality of medical services.

## 3.12 Other Systemic Diseases

Peng Wang and Kang-Yin Chen

AI-ECG has played an important role in the diagnosis of cardiovascular system diseases. At the same time, we can also see that AI-ECG has also achieved promising results in the identification and diagnosis of electrolyte disorders in the previous chapter. However, AI-ECG is not limited to only identifying heart disease. Traditional electrocardiographic research using indicators obtained from ECG, such as heart rate variability (HRV), has demonstrated good potential in the field of non-cardiac diseases such as epilepsy and obstructive sleep apnea syndrome. With the development of new algorithms such as deep learning, AI-ECG has made great achievements in patient information identification, physiological index measurement, auxiliary diagnosis of neuropsychiatric diseases and respiratory diseases, as well as drug safety monitoring. This chapter will start with the above-mentioned fields, exploring the diverse roles of AI-ECG and broadening the readers' interests toward AI-ECG.

### 3.12.1 AI-ECG and Personal Information Identification

Electrocardiographic studies have identified that different ages and genders display variable performances on ECG. Dutch scholars [199] analyzed the ECG of about 13,000 healthy individuals aged 16–90 years and showed that the heart rate-corrected trend of QT interval (QTc interval) and mean QRS axis will change with age. Taking QTc interval as an example, the median QTc interval of young males is 405 milliseconds, while the median of long males gradually approached 420 milliseconds. The upper limit remained in the range of 440–450 milliseconds, while the QTc interval climbed to 460 milliseconds in the 70–79 age group. Interestingly, it was even higher in people over 80 years old when examining gender. In addition to the conventional QTc interval, several studies have shown that the PQ interval [200], the QT/RR curvature [201], the interval from the J point to the end of the T wave, the interval from the J point to the peak of the T wave, and the interval from the end of the T wave (Tp-e interval) [202] also contained gender differences.

In recent years, some scholars have also used the above and other electrocardiographic indicators to predict the difference between the patient's ECG age and actual age [203], as well as the relationship with mortality [204], but the diagnostic efficiency is not high. For example, Japanese scholars [204] used approximately standard 12-lead ECG data from 19,000 patients of all ages excluding structural heart disease using principal component analysis (PCA) and obtained an age prediction model containing 438 ECG indicators. The highest attained AUC was only 0.731.

Attia et al. [205] used 774,783 standard 12-lead ECGs of adult patients to predict age and gender, and 499,727 standard 12-lead ECG samples of 10 s were used to train CNN. The trained algorithm was independently tested in the remaining cohort of 275,056 patients. For gender prediction, the algorithm achieved an AUC of 0.97 on the independent test data. For age prediction, the average error was 6.9 ± 5.6 years. The main factors for the age predicted by the algorithm were to be more than 7 years than the actual age included, as well as low ejection fraction, hypertension, and coronary heart disease ($P < 0.01$). This suggested that age predicted by AI-ECG may be associated with poor prognosis.

Lima et al. [206] further confirmed that the "ECG age" obtained by the AI-ECG algorithm can be used as a predictor of mortality. The research team used 1,558,415 cases (40.2% were male, with a mean age of 51.6 ± 17.6 years) of patient ECG data. 85% of the above cohorts were pre-divided as training datasets, and the remaining 15% and two other independent cohorts composed of 14,236 and 1631 patients were used as validation cohorts. The improved residual network was applied after the CNN algorithm had trained the model, obtaining the predicted value of "ECG age." The result of comparison with the actual age shows that in the 15% verification cohort set aside in advance, the "ECG age" of 8 years or older than the actual age showed patients had a higher risk of death (HR: 1.79, 95% CI: 1.69–1.90; $P < 0.001$). When their "ECG age" was 8 years younger than the actual age, the risk of death was lower (HR: 0.78, 95% CI: 0.74–0.83, P < 0.001). The verification results of the other two independent external cohorts were similar to those of the 15% verification cohort set aside in advance. It shows that "ECG age" plays a certain role in predicting the risk of death.

The German Strodthoff [207] team recently used the public PTB-XL dataset (including standard 10-s 12-lead ECGs from 18,885 patients) and the ICBEB 2018 dataset (including standard 12-lead ECGs from 6877 patients). Smaller-scale datasets, using different types of CNN algorithms, compare the effects of each algorithm in the field of gender and age prediction, among which the residual network xresnet1d101 performed best in the field of gender prediction, with an AUC of 0.92. The residual network resnet1d_wang also performed well in the field of age prediction, with a mean absolute error (MAE) of 6.9 years (coefficient of determination R2 = 0.7).

The above research results suggest that we can use AI-ECG in the field of age and gender prediction. Whether we can use gender and other clinical information to calibrate "ECG age" to make it more consistent with actual age or use "ECG age" to predict heart failure. The evaluation of treatment effects in patients is worthy of further study.

### 3.12.2 AI-ECG and Physiological Index Measurement

AI-ECG has shown great potential in the field of physiological index measurement. The AI algorithm simply analyzes the ECG and has advanced from the initial classification era of distinguishing the presence of an anomaly, such as whether the patient has high blood pressure and whether there is hypoglycemia at night. The machine can accurately provide specific measurement values, such as the measurement era of the patient's current blood pressure and glycosylated hemoglobin-specific values. This section will first explore blood pressure prediction and blood glucose monitoring and highlight recent advancements made by AI-ECG in the measurement of physiological indicators.

#### 3.12.2.1 AI-ECG and Blood Pressure Prediction

The existing cuff-type blood pressure measurement method can conveniently obtain the blood pressure value at a certain moment in the clinic or at home. However, if continuous blood pressure monitoring is required, ambulatory blood pressure monitoring may immobilize the patient. In addition, invasive blood pressure monitoring equipment is expensive. Invasive operation is not conducive to clinical promotion. Long-term hypertension can cause left ventricular hypertrophy, which is reflected in ECG as an increase in the Sokolow-Lyon index (the sum of the amplitude of the R wave in lead V5 and the absolute value of the amplitude of the S wave in lead V1) and other indicators. AI-ECG's prediction of blood pressure has undergone a transformation from simply distinguishing whether there is hypertension to outputting specific blood pressure values.

Rajput et al. [208, 209] used the feature extraction method to classify whether adverse events occurred in hypertensive patients. The team used the SHAREE dataset, including 24-h ECG data of 139 subjects, to classify patients with myocardial infarction, stroke, and syncope. Hypertensive patients were defined as the high-risk hypertension group, and those without the above-mentioned events were defined as the low-risk hypertension group. Using the optimal orthogonal wavelet filtering method (OWFB) [208] to extract the signal fractal dimension (SFD). The logarithmic energy (LOGE) feature identifies low-risk hypertension and high-risk hypertension groups, and its identification accuracy can reach 100%. While having high accuracy, we should also see that the relevant studies only differentiated adverse events, and the patient's ECG changes significantly when accompanied by these events.

Ni [210] of Northwestern Polytechnical University also used the public SHAREE data to distinguish whether the systolic blood pressure is higher than 160 mmHg by using the HRV changes in the nighttime ECG data. The time pyramid pooling method was used to reduce the feature dimension, applying multi-factor analysis of variance to filter relevant features, and establishing a hypertension identification model with relevant features. The overall accuracy rate was attained to be 95.1%.

Soh et al. used the SHAREE data and 18 normal 24-h ECG signals from the MIT-Beth Israel Hospital (MIT-BIH) normal sinus rhythm database and used CNN to develop a method to identify hypertension (blood pressure ≥ 140/90 mmHg). The accuracy of the algorithm reached 99.9% accuracy using the above data. Although the recognition accuracy of the above research is very high, the data used were limited. It is not known whether the recognition accuracy will be reduced when it is extended to external real-world data. The traditional method is very convenient and fast for instantaneous blood pressure measurement, which may limit the clinical value of new classification algorithms that simply identify the occurrence of hypertension.

The development of AI-ECG provides the possibility to predict the value of blood pressure by using ECG signal alone or in combination with other physiological signals, such as photoelectric capacitance (PPG). Simjanoska et al. [211] used ECG records from 51 patients to extract 3129 30-s ECG segments. The above data were divided into training set, verification set, and test set according to the ratio of 6:1:3. The researchers used seven machine learning algorithms, namely, K-nearest neighbor (KNN), decision tree J48 classification algorithm, Naive Bayes, support vector machine (SVM), random forest, guided aggregation, and boosting. The study developed a three-category model to distinguish normal blood pressure (<120/80 mmHg), high-normal blood pressure (120/80 to 139/89 mmHg), and hypertension (≥140/90 mmHg) and used random forest algorithm to construct three different regression models to estimate systolic blood pressure, diastolic blood pressure, and mean arterial pressure. After calibrating the model, the MAE for systolic blood pressure decreased to 7.72 mmHg, decreased to 9.45 mmHg for diastolic blood pressure, and decreased to 8.13 mmHg for mean arterial pressure.

Mousavi et al. [212] used the MIMIC II dataset (intensive care data containing single-lead II leads) to extract features from ECG using frequency domain analysis. Blood pressure values were then estimated using decision trees, neural networks, correlation vector regression, and random forest regression. The random forest algorithm had the lowest MAE, with a systolic blood pressure MAE of 12.75 mmHg, a diastolic blood pressure MAE of 6.04 mmHg, and a mean arterial blood pressure MAE of 7.01 mmHg. The above studies all used traditional machine learning related algorithms for learning, and the data has not been verified by real external data. Recently, Miao [163] of the Shenzhen Institute of Advanced Technology used the MIMIC III database (including the intensive care data of the single lead II lead of 1711 patients), and used a fusion model including the residual network and the long short-term memory network to construct blood pressure estimation. At the same time, the algorithm was verified in the external data composed of 30 patients in Fuwai Hospital in China. The results showed that the estimated errors of the predicted systolic blood pressure, mean arterial pressure and diastolic blood pressure, and the actual measured values were $-0.22 \pm 5.82$ mmHg, $-0.57 \pm 4.39$ mmHg, and $-0.75 \pm 5.62$ mmHg, respectively.

Another idea for AI-ECG to predict blood pressure is to use it with other physiological signals and clinical characteristics to increase the reliability and accuracy of the measurement results. PPG is most used in conjunction with ECG signals. The pulse wave arrival time (PAT) refers to the time interval between the R wave peak of ECG and the systolic peak of PPG. When the PAT is longer, it indicates that the patient's blood pressure is low. Yang et al. [213] collected ECG and PPG signals from 45 subjects and at the same time input their basic clinical characteristics (age, height, weight, and gender) together with the collected signals into a CNN and long short-term memory (in the fusion algorithm composed of LSTM) algorithm. The study results showed that the MAE of diastolic and systolic blood pressure predicted by the model were $3.23 \pm 4.75$ mmHg and $4.43 \pm 6.09$ mmHg, respectively.

Baker et al. [214] improved the fusion algorithm of CNN and LSTM by using the ECG signal and PPG signal data of the MIMIC III database. The results showed that the MAE of systolic blood pressure, diastolic blood pressure, and mean arterial pressure were 4.41 mmHg, 2.91 mmHg, and 2.77 mmHg, respectively. Sagirova et al. [215] integrated the developed algorithm combining ECG signal and PPG signal into the smartphone case, recruited 500 subjects, and tested the AI algorithm in the field. The measurement accuracy of blood pressure in real people shows that the error range of systolic blood pressure is $3.63 \pm 0.32$ mmHg, and the error range of diastolic blood pressure is $2.95 \pm 0.61$ mmHg.

In terms of blood pressure prediction, AI-ECG has developed rapidly from a simple classification algorithm, which has only scientific research value, to a prediction value comparable to the measurement results of a sphygmomanometer. This is a promising example demonstrating the potential of AI-ECG. However, there have been a small number of studies [215] that advanced the relevant algorithm into actual clinical application, and large-scale prospective non-inferiority clinical trials comparing the relationship between the relevant algorithm and the sphygmomanometer are worth further investigating.

#### 3.12.2.2 AI-ECG and Blood Glucose Monitoring

The difference between blood glucose monitoring and blood pressure testing is that blood pressure testing is non-invasive and can be done conveniently at home, while the existing blood glucose monitoring methods are all invasive procedures, thus affecting patient compliance. Previous electrocardiographic analysis of healthy subjects infused with insulin [216] showed that the hypoglycemia group had shortened PR interval, prolonged QTc interval, R wave amplitude, and area compared to the non-hypoglycemia group. In addition, the T wave amplitude and area were significantly decreased. A similar monitoring study of hypoglycemia in patients with type 1 diabetes mellitus (T1DM) [217] also found that the QTc interval was prolonged during hypoglycemia, suggesting that changes in blood sugar will cause corresponding changes in ECG, which provides a theoretical basis for follow-up AI-ECG blood glucose monitoring. At present, the research on AI-ECG and blood glucose monitoring mainly focuses on the early identification of hypoglycemia events or diabetes classification. Not only is the current blood glucose monitoring equipment invasive, but many patients with T1DM may often have hypoglycemia events at night. Hence, it is difficult to isolate hypoglycemic symptoms, so it is crucial to find a simple and accurate identification method.

Ling et al. [218] analyzed the ECG data of a 10-h nocturnal hypoglycemia study consisting of 16 children with T1DM (average age 14.6 ± 1.5 years). The researchers used a continuous blood glucose monitoring device to monitor each patient at night to understand the natural occurrence of nocturnal hypoglycemia. Hypoglycemia was defined as a blood glucose level less than 3.33 mmol/L, and severe hypoglycemia was defined as a blood glucose level less than 2.80 mmol/L. The researchers used the patient's heart rate and QTc interval to construct a fuzzy inference model mixed with particle swarm optimization. The results showed that the sensitivity of detecting severe hypoglycemia reached 85.71% and the specificity was 79.84%, but the sensitivity of hypoglycemic episodes was 80.00% while the specificity was only 55.14%. The research team [219] continued to improve the monitoring method for nocturnal hypoglycemia in children with T1DM by using the AI method. The team used the ECG data of a 10-h nocturnal hypoglycemia study of 15 children with T1DM to analyze. The nocturnal hypoglycemia blood sugar refers to blood sugar less than 3.33 mmol/L. This time, the researchers also inputted the patient's heart rate and QTc interval information into the deep belief network (DBN), block-based neural network (BBNN), and wavelet neural network (WNN). Different neural network models, such as feed-forward neural network (FFNN) and traditional multiple regression (MR) models, were compared to identify the effectiveness of different models for nocturnal hypoglycemia. The results showed that DBN had the best identification effect, with a sensitivity of 92.8%, although the attained specificity of 50% was still low.

The development of deep learning has made it possible to improve the recognition of hypoglycemia. Porumb et al. [220] tracked whether hypoglycemia events occurred during 14 nights of sleep in a small-scale study including only eight healthy subjects. At the same time, the 24-h dynamic ECG signals within 14 days were collected. Hypoglycemia was defined as a blood sugar level of less than 4.0 mmol/L. The researchers sent the collected ECG signals to the CNN and the joint algorithm of CNN and recurrent neural network (RNN), respectively. To compare the optimal recognition algorithm, the results show that the combined algorithm of CNN and RNN is the most robust, with a sensitivity of 84.7% and a specificity of 84.5%.

The monitoring of blood glucose by AI-ECG is not limited to the early identification of hypoglycemia at night. Some studies [221, 222] focused on the effect of AI-ECG on pre-diabetes [221] (impaired fasting blood glucose with or without glucose tolerance). The AI-ECG was used to predict the level of glycosylated hemoglobin following the concept of "ECG age," and the AI-ECG was used to predict the level of glycosylated hemoglobin [222]. "ECG glycosylated hemoglobin" was proposed to monitor the control of diabetes.

Wang et al. [221] used the standard 12-lead 5-s ECG data of 2914 subjects for analysis, of which 2251 subjects were used as the training set and 663 subjects were used as the test set. The study defined fasting blood glucose concentration to be between 6.1 and 6.9 mmol/L, as well as a blood glucose value of less than 7.8 mmol/L 2 h after an oral glucose tolerance test. Impaired glucose tolerance was defined as a fasting blood glucose level of less than 7.0 mmol/L and oral blood glucose to be between 7.8 and 11.1 mmol/L 2 h after the glucose tolerance test. The researchers developed a set of two-dimensional CNN algorithms called IGRNet, which included four convolutional layers, two pooling layers, a fully connected layer, and an output layer (input layer—convolutional layer—convolutional layer—pooling layer—convolutional layer—convolutional layer—pooling layer—fully connected layer—output layer). Because the input ECG data were all original images, the researchers used the micro-cropping method to slightly crop the ECG photo without adjusting its direction. This was to achieve the purpose of data augmentation and balance the samples. After data augmentation, researchers used histogram of oriented gradients (HOG) to extract ECG image features and input them into traditional machine learning models, such as SVM, random forest, and K nearest neighbors, for performance comparison among algorithms. The results showed that IGRNet had the highest diagnostic accuracy and AUC of 0.781 and 0.777, respectively.

Lin et al. [222] used 104,823 ECGs with traceable corresponding glycated hemoglobin and fasting blood glucose as the training set to train the algorithm to calculate the corresponding "ECG glycated hemoglobin," and 2190 ECGs provided by 1539 patients were used as the test set to evaluate the calculated "ECG." The difference between "glycosylated hemoglobin" and real glycated hemoglobin, as well as the ECG of another 3293 patients, were used to analyze the impact of "electrocardiogram-glycated hemoglobin" on diabetes. The researchers used a deep learning model including a residual module for training and testing, and the MAE of "ECG glycosylated hemoglobin" was 1.230. Prediction cohort results showed that during a median follow-up of 4.5 years, higher "ECG HbA1c" ("ECG HbA1c" > 6.5%) was associated with death (HR: 1.53, 95% CI: 1.08–2.17), new-onset chronic kidney disease heart failure (HR: 1.56, 95% CI: 1.30–1.87), and new-onset heart failure (HR: 1.51, 95% CI: 1.13–2.01), suggesting that "ECG glycosylated hemoglobin" may be a novel predictor of the prognosis of diabetes and its complications.

The monitoring of blood glucose by AI-ECG is still in its infancy, but the existing research is exciting for the non-invasive identification of nocturnal hypoglycemia and pre-diabetes, as well as predicting the level of glycosylated hemoglobin. Non-invasive blood sugar identification devices are on the rise. Non-commercialized medical-grade non-invasive blood glucose recognition devices have been put on the market, and AI-ECG is expected to play more pioneering roles in blood glucose monitoring.

### 3.12.3 AI-ECG and Auxiliary Diagnosis of Nervous and Mental Diseases

HRV is regulated by the sympathetic and parasympathetic nervous systems, and emotional changes will affect the body's sympathetic and parasympathetic nervous systems, thereby indirectly affecting HRV [223]. So can we use relevant changes to capture changes in people's nervous systems from ECG? Some studies focus on this, and at the same time, it is possible to explore related fields by using AI-ECG methods. The following will discuss the feasibility of AI-ECG to decipher the perspective of the general public on AI-ECG's identification of nervous system and mental system diseases.

#### 3.12.3.1 AI-ECG and Auxiliary Diagnosis of Nervous System Diseases

AI-ECG's assisted identification of neurological diseases is mainly concentrated in the field of epilepsy and Parkinson's. The onset of such diseases seriously affects the quality of life of patients, so early identification and diagnosis are imperative. Taking epilepsy as an example, the traditional EEG monitoring method requires professional venues and personnel, which is not conducive to automatic detection, while the existing portable ECG monitoring device can realize long-term monitoring without affecting the patient's rest.

Cooman [224] et al. conducted a total of 918 h of single-lead (Lead II) monitoring on 17 patients with refractory temporal lobe epilepsy, recorded a total of 127 grand mal seizures, and then extracted the heart rate characteristic information from the ECG, which was input into the SVM algorithm. The results showed that the recognition accuracy of the algorithm for temporal lobe grand mal seizures was 81.89%. Yamak [225] conducted a small-scale exploratory verification of the predictive effect of the ECG monitoring device developed by him on seven patients with refractory epilepsy. It consists of a smartphone that receives ECG data. The collected ECG signals are subjected to feature extraction to obtain relevant time domain and frequency domain features, and then inputted into the multivariate statistical process control (MSPC) algorithm to test the algorithm's prediction of epileptic seizures. The results show that the sensitivity of the relevant algorithm is 85.7% within 15 minutes before the seizure, and the false alarm rate is 0.62 times per hour.

Akbilgic et al. [226] used standard 12-lead 10-second ECG data from 60 participants in the Honolulu-Asian Aging Study (HAAS). Among them, 10 participants were diagnosed with Parkinson's disease before ECG recording, 25 participants showed no evidence of Parkinson's disease during ECG recording but were diagnosed with Parkinson's disease during the 5-year follow-up period, and the remaining 25 participants were Parkinson-free throughout the follow-up period. The researchers first identified the R-peak for subsequent calculation of heart rate characteristics and used various methods, including fast Fourier transform (FFT), signal complexity, approximate entropy method with different parameter settings, and probabilistic symbolic pattern recognition (PSPR), to extract 794 kinds of ECG features. Then, the information was inputted into the stepwise logistic regression model. The results showed that the average AUC of the final regression model after fivefold cross-validation was 0.835 (95% CI: 0.831–0.839).

The sample size of AI-ECG in the field of the nervous system is relatively small, and it is still in its infancy. Due to the small sample size, researchers mostly use feature extraction combined with traditional machine learning algorithms with limited external verification. Deep learning often requires large-scale data as support, and we look forward to the fruition of combining ECG with deep learning.

#### 3.12.3.2 AI-ECG and Auxiliary Diagnosis of Mental Diseases

Turning to the field of psychiatric conditions, researchers have a wider range of interests, including bipolar disorder, post-traumatic stress disorder, and autism.

Gentili et al. [227] studied the ECG data of eight patients with bipolar disorder. The purpose of the study was to determine whether the AI-ECG method could distinguish the emotional state of patients with bipolar disorder. Physiological monitoring of patients with bipolar disorder with a wearable system from the Physiological Monitoring System (PSYCHE). The PSYCHE platform consists of T-shirts with wearable sensors and electrodes embedded in fabrics, which can be used to obtain ECG, respiratory signals, and physical activity information. Smartphones were also used to collect data from wearable systems via Bluetooth technology, which can be used to record voice parameters and subjective data (such as the emotional state involved in this study). The judgment of the specific emotional state is based on the scores of the Youth Mania Rating Scale (YMRS) and the Quick Inventory of Depressive Symptoms (QIDS-C): YMRS greater than 6 indicates a hypomanic state; QIDS-C greater than 8 indicates a depressed state. A bipolar state is considered if both scales exceed the aforementioned cutoff values. The researchers collected a total of 39 ECG recordings with a total duration of more than 300 h, including 11 hypomanic states, 13 depressive states, 2 bipolar states, and 13 normal states. After feature extraction, the above ECG data was extracted to obtain the corresponding time domain, frequency domain, and nonlinear domain features, and then inputted into SVM to construct the emotion recognition algorithm. The results showed that when the SVM was used to measure the emotional state of the patient before and after, the classification accuracy was up to 99.25%.

Reinertsen et al. [228] used the ECG information of 60 participants in the Emory Twin Study [229] to study whether the AI algorithm could correctly distinguish post-traumatic stress disorder. Of the 60 participants, 24 experienced typical PTSD symptoms within the past month, and the other 26 were healthy controls. All study participants recorded 24-h ambulatory ECGs using Holter. Due to the small sample size, researchers also used feature extraction methods to feed into machine learning algorithms. The researchers extracted a total of 20 features for training the logistic regression algorithm based on L1/L2 regularization, and the results showed that the AUC of the related algorithm was 0.87.

Frasch et al. [230] used the 5-minute ECG data of 69 child participants between the ages of 8 and 12 years to judge the effect of relevant machine learning algorithms on autism discrimination. In the study, 18 children with autism were considered children with conduct problems, 15 children were depressed, and 18 children were on a typical developmental path. The researchers also used the feature extraction method to extract relevant heart rate features and input them into the extreme gradient boosting (XGBoost) algorithm at a ratio of 8:2 between the training group and the test group. The results showed that the AUC of the XGBoost algorithm reached 0.89.

From the above studies, we can see that AI-ECG has been actively explored by various research teams in the early diagnosis of neurological and psychiatric diseases but is limited by the lack of high-quality large-scale databases. Current research often uses feature extraction methods as input for the machine learning algorithm. Notably, there is room for development in the application of deep learning in this field, and we also expect AI-ECG to make corresponding contributions in the diagnosis and treatment of stroke and more common diseases such as depression.

### 3.12.4 AI-ECG and Auxiliary Diagnosis of Respiratory Diseases

The application of AI-ECG to respiratory diseases mainly focuses on the diagnosis of obstructive sleep apnea syndrome. Polysomnography is considered the gold standard for the diagnosis of obstructive sleep apnea syndrome. However, its operation needs to be worn all night. Although some portable polysomnography devices have appeared, these corresponding devices still affect the sleep quality of patients to a certain extent. Alternative methods for diagnosing obstructive sleep apnea syndrome simply and conveniently have become a research hotspot.

The relationship between ECG and obstructive sleep apnea syndrome has been discovered long ago. HRV changes significantly during sleep apnea. As early as the end of the last century, ECG has been used in the diagnosis of obstructive sleep apnea syndrome [231]. Since the twenty-first century, the PhysioNet Apnea-ECG database, a public database containing ECG signals related to sleep apnea, has been frequently used. This database contains 70–100 Hz single-lead ECG signals, and each signal records ECG and blood oxygen saturation information of patients with obstructive sleep apnea syndrome and healthy controls during sleep for about 7–10 h. A total of 15 records were from healthy subjects, and the other 55 records were from patients with sleep apnea. The database provider even thoughtfully pre-designed a 1:1 training dataset and testing dataset in the database so that relevant researchers can conduct internal verification quickly. Researchers used feature extraction combined with traditional machine learning algorithms to perform the extraction. The relevant monitoring algorithm literature has been overwhelming [232]. In recent years, with the continuous development of deep learning, the accuracy of monitoring sleep apnea using ECG signals has reached a new level. Due to space limitations, this section mainly introduces the application of ECG deep learning technology in sleep apnea.

Wang et al. [233] used the PhysioNet Apnea-ECG database mentioned above to propose a sleep apnea detection framework based on CNN. The researchers first extracted the RR intervals from the ECG signals recorded in the database and then input the extracted RR intervals into the CNN model. The designed CNN model has three convolutional layers: The first two convolutional layers are followed by a batch normalization layer and max pooling layer; the third convolutional layer is followed by three fully connected layers; and the last fully connected layer is connected with a normalized index classifier to make a final decision to determine whether the ECG signal is from obstructive sleep apnea. The results of the study show that the final sensitivity, specificity, and overall accuracy of the model reached 100%, 93%, and 97.8% in the internal validation data. It is worth noting that, similar to many traditional machine learning methods, due to the relative lack of external verification data, whether the sensitivity of related algorithms can maintain a perfect score of 100% when they are extended to the real world, needs further verification.

The research of Mashrur et al. [234] provides the possibility for us to understand whether the algorithm obtained in the PhysioNet Apnea-ECG database can be extended to other data with the same ultra-high sensitivity. The researchers also used the PhysioNet Apnea-ECG database and utilized continuous wavelet transform (CWT) and empirical mode decomposition (EMD) to convert the ECG signal into a mixed scale map, which was then inputted into the mixed scale map. These scale maps are modeled in a lightweight CNN model to extract deep features for sleep apnea detection to determine whether the relevant ECG signal comes from a sleep apnea event. The results show that the relevant algorithm analyzing the PhysioNet Apnea-ECG dataset achieved an accuracy of 94.30%, sensitivity of 94.30%, and specificity of 94.51%. External validation using the correlation algorithm achieved an accuracy, sensitivity, and specificity of 78.96%, 68.19%, and 83.33%, respectively. It can be seen that in the external data, the accuracy of the relevant algorithms has declined significantly, which suggests that we need to carefully evaluate the algorithms before and during the application to meet the specific needs of different application scenarios.

The work of Mukherjee et al. [235] showed the possibility of integration between different algorithms and gave a preliminary answer for how to adjust related algorithms in the real world. The researchers segmented the ECG signals in the PhysioNet Apnea-ECG database every 1 min and obtained 15,961 and 15,938 samples in the training dataset and test dataset, respectively. Within the training set, there were 9832 sleep apnea samples and 6129 normal samples, while the test set had 9838 sleep apnea samples and 6100 normal samples. After further extracting the RR interval-related features from the above data, three different deep learning models were used for algorithm integration research, two of which were CNN-based models and a combination of CNN and LSTM fusion models. The researchers fed the above three deep learning models into four ensemble methods: majority voting, summation rule, Choquet integral-based fuzzy fusion, and trainable ensemble using a multilayer perceptron (MLP), and the results are shown in internal validation. The MLP-based ensemble method has the highest accuracy of 85.58% in the data. Although the overall accuracy has not been verified by external data, the accuracy of the integrated method was higher than that of the first three deep learning models without integration. This may provide a feasible solution for improving the accuracy of the algorithm in external data.

The application of AI-ECG in respiratory diseases, especially sleep apnea syndrome, fully reflects the advantages of data. With the help of the public PhysioNet Apnea-ECG database, researchers can fully test the pros and cons of different techniques. At the same time, it is hoped that more research will focus on external data validation because existing research suggests that the high accuracy achieved by the algorithm in the internal test dataset may not be ideal in external data. In reality, close communication between medical staff and algorithm engineers may produce an unexpected inspiration train of thought.

### 3.12.5 AI-ECG and Medication Safety Monitoring

The existing drug safety monitoring mainly consists of the adverse reaction reporting system after the drug is marketed and the blood drug concentration monitoring during hospitalization. The adverse reaction reporting system has a corresponding lag, and the blood drug concentration monitoring requires the close cooperation of the pharmaceutical team. The drugs often used by cardiologists may have adverse effects on the heart itself in a small probability. For example, anti-arrhythmic drugs themselves have arrhythmogenic effects. The toxic dose is very close, and how to early monitor the impact of related drugs on the heart has become a topic of concern to cardiologists and pharmaceutical professionals.

The emergence of AI-ECG has provided a new perspective for solving the above problems. Several small-scale exploratory AI-ECG [187, 236, 237] studies focusing on the effect of drugs on the QT interval have made it possible to monitor preventive drugs only by ECG.

Dofetilide is a class III antiarrhythmic drug that produces anti-arrhythmic effects by blocking potassium ion channels and can be used to control a variety of arrhythmias. Prolonging the QT interval may induce Torsades de pointes. The following two small-scale studies use AI methods to provide a reference for the non-invasive detection of dofetilide blood concentration through ECG signals. Attia et al. [187] obtained data from standard 12-lead 10-s ECG and explored it in relation to the plasma concentration of fetilide. One of the studies aimed to compare the ECG effects of dofetilide, quinidine, ranolazine, and verapamil on healthy subjects, including 22 subjects who received dofetilide [238]. Another study aimed to reveal the effect of mexiletine, lidocaine, and diltiazem on the QT interval of patients receiving dofetilide or moxifloxacin [239], including information of 20 patients who received dofetilide treatment. The researchers divided the above 42 subjects into a training set composed of 30 subjects and a test set composed of 12 patients. The researchers developed a set with an unsupervised CNN model with seven convolutional layers and two fully connected layers to predict the blood concentration of dofetilide. This was compared with the traditional linear regression model generated by the QTc interval calculated by the Bazett method. The results show that the unsupervised CNN model prediction (correlation coefficient r = 0.85) was significantly better than the traditional QTc model (r = 0.64). Morettini et al. [236] used the aforementioned study involving 22 subjects to compare the ECG effects of dofetilide, quinidine, ranolazine, and verapamil on healthy subjects [238]. The feature extraction method was used to obtain T wave-related features on ECG, and the data were inputted into the artificial neural network model (ANN) to predict whether QT interval prolongation occurs. The results show that the correlation algorithm has a high predictive value in QT prolongation, and the AUC reached 0.91.

The public's attention to the QT interval is not limited to dofetilide. Maille et al. [237] used the developed AI algorithm to predict the QTc interval and evaluated the single-guidance data recorded by the smartwatch in 85 subjects. Due to the consistency of the measurement of QTc interval between the ECG signal and the standard 12-lead ECG, the above-mentioned subjects received hydroxychloroquine combined with azithromycin for the treatment of new coronary pneumonia. However, the above-mentioned therapy may lead to prolongation of the QTc interval, and there is a potential to induce Torsade ventricular tachycardia. The researchers recorded the standard 12-lead ECG at the time of enrollment, on the sixth and tenth days of the study, and based on this to judge the predictive value of the smartwatch on the QTc interval. Although the above scheme has been confirmed to be unhelpful for the treatment of new coronary pneumonia [240], the study showed that the QTc interval predicted by the smartwatch and the results calculated by the standard 12-lead ECG have a good consistency. In 98.2% of the patients, the difference between the measured values is less than 50 ms.

Another study [241] applied AI-ECG to the detection of digoxin toxicity. Since the effective blood concentration of digoxin is close to the toxic dose, using AI-ECG to identify early digoxin poisoning can avoid invasive blood drug concentration monitoring. Subsequently, this can reduce the psychological and economic burden on patients. Chang et al. [240] collected 61 ECGs of 34 cases of digoxin poisoning and the remaining 177,066 other ECGs into the artificial learning algorithm. Digoxin poisoning was defined as blood drug concentration greater than or equal to 2 ng/mL, and the ratio of training set to test set was 8:2. The researchers developed an 82-layer CNN called ECG12Net, and the results showed that the related algorithm achieved an AUC of 0.912 in the test set and an AUC of 0.929 in the human-computer comparison.

The application of AI-ECG in drug safety is still in the exploratory stage. Existing research focuses on the safety monitoring of antiarrhythmic drugs and cardiac drugs that have a significant impact on the heart. At the same time, we have reason to expect AI-ECG to fight against tumors. It plays a more active role in the cardiotoxicity of drugs and even expands to the field of safety monitoring of more types of drugs.

### 3.12.6 Prospects and Prospects

AI-ECG has greatly broadened the scope of application of ECG, and many ideas that were considered unconstrained in the past are gradually being transformed into research with practical application value and clinical transformation space. Many applications, such as gender and age, blood pressure measurement, and sleep apnea syndrome judgment, have a certain electrocardiological basis. AI has the advantage of analyzing massive data and can discover connections that the human eye could not find in the past. In the future, we look forward to further research on AI algorithms and make more efforts to open the invisible "black box," so as to achieve the effect that clinicians know and trust AI.

## References


1. Al'Aref SJ, Anchouche K, Singh G, et al. Clinical applications of machine learning in cardiovascular disease and its relevance to cardiac imaging. Eur Heart J. 2019;40(24):1975–86.
2. Antoniades C, Asselbergs FW, Vardas P. The year in cardiovascular medicine 2020: digital health and innovation. Eur Heart J. 2021;42(7):732–9.
3. Siontis KC, Noseworthy PA, Attia ZI, et al. Artificial intelligence-enhanced electrocardiography in cardiovascular disease management. Nat Rev Cardiol. 2021;18(7):465–78.
4. Quer G, Muse ED, Topol EJ, et al. Long data from the electrocardiogram. Lancet. 2019;393:10187.
5. Krittanawong C, Kaplin S. Artificial intelligence in global health. Eur Heart J. 2021;42(24):2321–2.
6. Bax JJ, van der Bijl P, Delgado V. Machine learning for electrocardiographic diagnosis of left ventricular early diastolic dysfunction. J Am Coll Cardiol. 2018;71(15):1661–2.
7. Sengupta PP, Kulkarni H, Narula J. Prediction of abnormal myocardial relaxation from signal processed surface ECG. J Am Coll Cardiol. 2018;71(15):1650–60.
8. Attia ZI, Kapa S, Lopez Jimenez F, et al. Screening for cardiac contractile dysfunction using an artificial intelligence-enabled electrocardiogram. Nat Med. 2019;25(1):70–4.
9. Kagiyama N, Piccirilli M, Yanamala N, et al. Machine learning assessment of left ventricular diastolic function based on electrocardiographic features. J Am Coll Cardiol. 2020;76(8):930–41.
10. Attia ZI, Noseworthy PA, Lopez-Jimenez F, et al. An artificial intelligence-enabled ECG algorithm for the identification of patients with atrial fibrillation during sinus rhythm: a retrospective analysis of outcome prediction. Lancet. 2019;394(10201):861–7.
11. Hendriks JML, Fabritz L. AI can now identify atrial fibrillation through sinus rhythm. Lancet. 2019;394(10201):812–3.
12. Wolters FJ. An AI-ECG algorithm for atrial fibrillation risk: steps towards clinical implementation. Lancet. 2020;396(10246):235–6.
13. Hannun AY, Rajpurkar P, Haghpanahi M, et al. Cardiologist-level arrhythmia detection and classification in ambulatory electrocardiograms using a deep neural network. Nat Med. 2019;25(1):65–9.
14. Ribeiro AH, Ribeiro MH, Paixao GMM, et al. Automatic diagnosis of the 12-lead ECG using a deep neural network. Nat Commun. 2020;11(1):1760.
15. Al-Zaiti S, Besomi L, Bouzid Z, et al. Machine learning-based prediction of acute coronary syndrome using only the pre-hospital 12-lead electrocardiogram. Nat Commun. 2020;11(1):3966.
16. Ko WY, Siontis KC, Attia ZI, et al. Detection of hypertrophic cardiomyopathy using a convolutional neural network-enabled electrocardiogram. J Am Coll Cardiol. 2020;75(7):722–33.
17. Tison GH, Zhang J, Delling FN, et al. Automated and interpretable patient ECG profiles for disease detection, tracking, and discovery. Circ Cardiovasc Qual Outcomes. 2019;12(9):e005289.
18. Goto S, Mahara K, Beussink-Nelson L, et al. Artificial intelligence-enabled fully automated detection of cardiac amyloidosis using electrocardiograms and echocardiograms. Nat Commun. 2021;12(1):2726.

19. Galloway CD, Valys AV, Shreibati JB, et al. Development and validation of a deep-learning model to screen for hyperkalemia from the electrocardiogram. JAMA Cardiol. 2019;4(5):428–36.
20. Cohen-Shelly M, Attia ZI, Friedman PA, et al. Electrocardiogram screening for aortic valve stenosis using artificial intelligence. Eur Heart J. 2021;42(30):2885–96.
21. Donal E, Hubert A, Le Rolle V, et al. New multiparametric analysis of cardiac dyssynchrony: machine learning and prediction of response to CRT. JACC Cardiovasc Imaging. 2019;12(9):1887–8.
22. Feeny AK, Rickard J, Trulock KM, et al. Machine learning of 12-lead QRS waveforms to identify cardiac resynchronization therapy patients with differential outcomes. Circ Arrhythm Electrophysiol. 2020;13(7):e008210.
23. Zhao Y, Xiong J, Hou Y, et al. Early detection of ST-segment elevated myocardial infarction by artificial intelligence with 12-lead electrocardiogram. Int J Cardiol. 2020;317:223–30.
24. Makimoto H, Hockmann M, Lin T, et al. Performance of a convolutional neural network derived from an ECG database in recognizing myocardial infarction. Sci Rep. 2020;10(1):8445.
25. Cho Y, Kwon JM, Kim KH, et al. Artificial intelligence algorithm for detecting myocardial infarction using six-lead electrocardiography. Sci Rep. 2020;10(1):20495.
26. Giudicessi JR, Schram M, Bos JM, et al. Artificial intelligence-enabled assessment of the heart rate corrected QT interval using a Mobile electrocardiogram device. Circulation. 2021;143(13):1274–86.
27. Somani S, Russak AJ, Richter F, et al. Deep learning and the electrocardiogram: review of the current state-of-the-art. Europace. 2021;23(8):1179–91.
28. Corral-Acero J, Margara F, Marciniak M, et al. The'digital twin' to enable the vision of precision cardiology. Eur Heart J. 2020;41(48):4556–64.
29. Yao X, McCoy RG, Friedman PA, et al. ECG AI-Guided Screening for Low Ejection Fraction(EAGLE): rationale and design of a pragmatic cluster randomized trial. Am Heart J. 2020;219:31–6.
30. Yao X, Rushlow DR, Inselman JW, et al. Artificial intelligence-enabled electrocardio-grams for identification of patients with low ejection fraction: a pragmatic, randomized clinical trial. Nat Med. 2021;27(5):815–9.
31. The Writing Committee of the Report on Cardiovascular Health and Diseases in China. Report on cardiovascular health and diseases burden in China: an updated summary of 2020. Chin Circul J. 2021;36(6):521–45.
32. Davari Dolatabadi A, Khadem SEZ, Asl BM. Automated diagnosis of coronary artery disease (CAD) patients using optimized SVM. Comput Methods Prog Biomed. 2017;138:117–26.
33. Patidar S, Pachori RB, Acharya UR. Automated diagnosis of coronary artery disease usingtunable-Q wavelet transform applied on heart rate signals. Knowl-Based Syst. 2015;82:1–10.
34. Butun E, Yildirim O, Talo M, et al. 1D-CADCapsNet: one dimensional deep capsule networks for coronary artery disease detection using ECG signals. Phys Med. 2020;70:39–48.
35. Jahmunah V, Ng EYK, San TR, et al. Automated detection of coronary artery disease,myocardial infarction and congestive heart failure using GaborCNN model with ECG signals. Comput Biol Med. 2021;134:104457.
36. Lih OS, Jahmunah V, San TR, et al. Comprehensive electrocardiographic diagnosis basedon deep learning. Artif Intell Med. 2020;103:101789.
37. Liu W, Zhang M, Zhang Y, et al. Real-time multilead convolutional neural network for myocardial infarction detection. IEEE J Biomed Health Inform. 2018;22(5):1434–44.
38. Al-Zaiti S, Besomi L, Bouzid Z, et al. Machine learning-based prediction of acute coronary syndrome using only the pre-hospital 12-lead electrocardiogram. Nat Commun. 2020;11(1):3966.
39. Liu WC, Lin CS, Tsai CS, et al. A deep-learning algorithm for detecting acute myocardial infarction. EuroIntervention. 2021;17(9):765–73.

40. Chen X, Guo W, Zhao L, et al. Acute myocardial infarction detection using deep learning-enabled electrocardiograms. Front Cardiovasc Med. 2021;8:654515.
41. Hussein AF, Hashim SJ, Rokhani FZ, et al. An automated high-accuracy detection scheme for myocardial ischemia based on multi-Lead long-interval ECG and Choi-Williams time-frequency analysis incorporating a multi-class SVM classifier. Sensors (Basel). 2021;21(7):2311.
42. Fernandez Biscay C, Arini PD, Rincon Soler AI, et al. Classification of ischemic and non-ischemic cardiac events in Holter recordings based on the continuous wavelettransform. Med Biol Eng Comput. 2020;58(5):1069–78.
43. Gumpfer N, Grun D, Hannig J, et al. Detecting myocardial scar using electrocardiogramdata and deep neural networks. Biol Chem. 2021;402(8):911–23.
44. Wang HM, Zhao W, Jia DY, et al. Myocardial infarction detection based on multi-lead ensemble neural network. Annu Int Conf IEEE Eng Med Biol Soc. 2019;2019:2614–7.
45. Zeng W, Yuan J, Yuan C, et al. Classification of myocardial infarction based on hybrid feature extraction and artificial intelligence tools by adopting tunable-Q wavelet transform (TQWT), variational mode decomposition(VMD)and neural networks. Artif Intell Med. 2020;106:101848.
46. Fu L, Lu B, Nie B, et al. Hybrid network with attention mechanism for detection and location of myocardial infarction based on 12-lead electrocardiogram signals. Sensors (Basel). 2020;20(4):1020.
47. Sharma M, Tan RS, Acharya UR. A novel automated diagnostic system for classificationof myocardial infarction ECG signals using an optimal biorthogonal filter bank. Comput Biol Med. 2018;102:341–56.
48. Ponikowski P, Voors AA, Anker SD, et al. 2016 ESC Guidelines for the diagnosis and treatment of acute and chronic heart failure: The Task Force for the diagnosis and treatment ofacute and chronic heart failure of the European Society of Cardiology(ESC). Developed with thespecial contribution of the Heart Failure Association (HFA) of the ESC. Eur J Heart Fail. 2016;18(8):891–975.
49. Heart Failure Group of Chinese Society of Cardiology of Chinese Medical Association, Chinese Heart Failure Association of Chinese Medical Doctor Association, Editorial Board of Chinese Journal of Cardiology. Chinese guidelines for the diagnosis and treatment of heart failure 2018. Chin J Cardiol. 2018;46(10):760–89.
50. Ponikowski P, Anker SD, AlHabib KF, et al. Heart failure: preventing disease and death worldwide. ESC Heart Fail. 2014;1(1):4–25.
51. Lund LH, Savarese G. Global public health burden of heart failure. Card Fail Rev. 2017;3(1):7–11.
52. Melillo P, Fusco R, Sansone M, et al. Discrimination power of long-term heart rate variability measures for chronic heart failure detection. Med Biol Eng Comput. 2011;49(1):67–74.
53. Zhang Y, Yang Q, Pang W, et al. Congestive heart failure detection via short-time electrocardiographic monitoring for fast reference advice in urgent medical conditions. Annu Int Conf IEEE Eng Med Biol Soc. 2018;2018:2256–9.
54. Liu G, Wang L, Wang Q, et al. A new approach to detect congestive heart failure using short-term heart rate variability measures. PLoS One. 2014;9(4):e93399.
55. Wang L, Zhou X. Detection of congestive heart failure based on LSTM-based deep network via short-term RR intervals. Sensors (Basel). 2019;19(7):1502.
56. Masetic Z, Subasi A. Congestive heart failure detection using random forest classifier. Comput Methods Prog Biomed. 2016;130:54–64.
57. Acharya UR, Fujita H, Oh SL, et al. Deep convolutional neural network for the automated diagnosis of congestive heart failure using ECG signals. Appl Intell. 2018;49(1):16–27.
58. Cho J, Lee B, Kwon JM, et al. Artificial intelligence algorithm for screening heart failure with reduced ejection fraction using electrocardiography. ASAIO J. 2021;67(3):314–21.
59. Chiou YA, Hung CL, Lin SF. AI-assisted echocardiographic prescreening of heart failure with preserved ejection fraction on the basis of intrabeat dynamics. JACC Cardiovasc Imaging. 2021;14(11):2091–104.

60. Kwon JM, Kim KH, Jeon KH, et al. Development and validation of deep-learning algorithm for electrocardiography-based heart failure identification. Korean Circ J. 2019;49(7):629–39.
61. Cinar A, Tuncer SA. Classification of normal sinus rhythm, abnormal arrhythmia and congestive heart failure ECG signals using LSTM and hybrid CNN-SVM deep neural networks. Comput Methods Biomech Biomed Engin. 2021;24(2):203–14.
62. U.S Food & Drug Administration. Fact sheet for patients emergency use of the ELEFT during the COVID-19 pandemic [DB/OL]. 2020.
63. Fathieh F, Paak M, Khosousi A, et al. Predicting cardiac disease from interactions of simultaneously-acquired hemodynamic and cardiac signals. Comput Methods Prog Biomed. 2021;202:105970.
64. Jentzer JC, Kashou AH, Attia ZI, et al. Left ventricular systolic dysfunction identificationusing artificial intelligence-augmented electrocardiogram in cardiac intensive care unit patients. Int J Cardiol. 2021;326:114–23.
65. Kashou AH, Noseworthy PA, Lopez-Jimenez F, et al. The effect of cardiac rhythm on artificial intelligence-enabled ECG evaluation of left ventricular ejection fraction prediction in cardiac intensive care unit patients. Int J Cardiol. 2021;339:54–5.
66. Davies RH, Jones AR. Machine learning for ECG diagnosis of LV dysfunction. JACC Cardiovasc Imaging. 2021;14(10):1916–7.
67. Potter EL, Rodrigues CHM, Ascher DB, et al. Machine learning of ECG waveforms to improve selection for testing for asymptomatic left ventricular dysfunction prompt. JACC Cardiovasc Imaging. 2021;4(10):1904–15.
68. Yao X, Rushlow DR, Inselman JW, et al. Artificial intelligence-enabled electrocardiograms for identification of patients with low ejection fraction: a pragmatic, randomized clinical trial. Nat Med. 2021;27(5):815–9.
69. Flachskampf FA, Biering-Sørensen T, Solomon SD, et al. Cardiac imaging to evaluate left ventricular diastolic function. JACC Cardiovasc Imaging. 2015;8(9):1071–93.
70. AlJaroudi WA, Thomas JD, Rodriguez LL, et al. Prognostic value of diastolic dysfunction: state of the art review. Cardiol Rev. 2014;22(2):79–90.
71. Khurshid S, Friedman S, Pirruccello JP, et al. Deep learning to predict cardiac magnetic resonance-derived left ventricular mass and hypertrophy from 12-lead ECGs. Circ Cardiovasc Imaging. 2021;14(6):e012281.
72. Cummings ED, Swoboda HD. Digoxin toxicity[M]. StatPearls Publishing LLC; 2021.
73. Chang DW, Lin CS, Tsao TP, et al. Detecting digoxin toxicity by artificial intelligence-assisted electrocardiography. Int J Environ Res Public Health. 2021;18(7):3839.
74. Tse G, Zhou J, Woo SWD, et al. Multi-modality machine learning approach for risk stratification in heart failure with left ventricular ejection fraction </= 45. ESC Heart Fail. 2020;7(6):3716–25.
75. Pandey A, Kagiyama N, Yanamala N, et al. Deep-learning models for the echocardiographic assessment of diastolic dysfunction. JACC Cardiovasc Imaging. 2021;14(10):1887–900. https://doi.org/10.1016/j.jcmg.2021.
76. Ortiz J, Ghefter CG, Silva CE, et al. One-year mortality prognosis in heart failure: a neural network approach based on echocardiographic data. J Am Coll Cardiol. 1995;26(7):1586–93.
77. Bazoukis G, Stavrakis S, Zhou J, et al. Machine learning versus conventional clinical methods in guiding management of heart failure patients-a systematic review. Heart Fail Rev. 2021;26(1):23–34.
78. Frizzell JD, Liang L, Schulte PJ, et al. Prediction of 30-day all-cause readmissions in patients hospitalized for heart failure: comparison of machine learning and other statistical approaches. JAMA Cardiol. 2017;2(2):204–9.
79. Awan SE, Bennamoun M, Sohel F, et al. Machine learning-based prediction of heart failure readmission or death: implications of choosing the right model and the right metrics. ESCHeart Fail. 2019;6(2):428–35.
80. Negassa A, Ahmed S, Zolty R, et al. Prediction model using machine learning for mortality in patients with heart failure. Am J Cardiol. 2021;153:86–93.

81. Jing L, Ulloa Cerna AE, Good CW, et al. A machine learning approach to managementof heart failure populations. JACC Heart Fail. 2020;8(7):578–87.
82. McNallan SM, Chamberlain AM, Gerber Y, et al. Measuring frailty in heart failure: a community perspective. Am Heart J. 2013;166(4):768–74.
83. Ju C, Zhou J, Lee S, et al. Derivation of an electronic frailty index for predicting short-term mortality in heart failure: a machine learning approach. ESC Heart Fail. 2021;8(4):2837–45.
84. Rawshani A, Rawshani A, Franzen S, et al. Risk factors, mortality, and cardiovascular outcomes in patients with type 2 diabetes. N Engl J Med. 2018;379(7):633–44.
85. Segar MW, Vaduganathan M, Patel KV, et al. Machine learning to predict the risk of incident heart failure hospitalization among patients with diabetes: the WATCH-DM risk score. Diabetes Care. 2019;42(12):2298–306.
86. Abraham WT, Adamson PB, Bourge RC, et al. Wireless pulmonary artery haemodynamicmonitoring in chronic heart failure: a randomised controlled trial. Lancet. 2011;377(9766):658–66.
87. Stehlik J, Schmalfuss C, Bozkurt B, et al. Continuous wearable monitoring analytics predict heart failure hospitalization: the LINK-HF multicenter study. Circ Heart Fail 2020;13(3):e006513.
88. Maron BJ, Towbin JA, Thiene G, et al. Contemporary definitions and classificationof the cardiomyopathies: an American Heart Association Scientific Statement from the Council onClinical Cardiology, Heart Failure and Transplantation Committee; Quality of Care and OutcomesResearch and Functional Genomics and Translational Biology Interdisciplinary Working Groups;and Council on Epidemiology and Prevention. Circulation. 2006;113(14):1807–16.
89. Maron BJ, Haas TS, Murphy CJ, et al. Incidence and causes of sudden death in U.S. college athletes. J Am Coll Cardiol. 2014;63(16):1636–43.
90. Ommen SR, Maron BJ, Olivotto I, et al. Long-term effects of surgical septal myectomy on survival in patients with obstructive hypertrophic cardiomyopathy. J Am Coll Cardiol. 2005;46(3):470–6.
91. Shrivastava S, Cohen-Shelly M, Attia ZI, et al. Artificial intelligence-enabled electrocardiography to screen patients with dilated cardiomyopathy. Am J Cardiol. 2021;155:121.
92. Attia ZI, Kapa S, Lopez-Jimenez F, et al. Screening for cardiac contractile dysfunction using an artificial intelligence-enabled electrocardiogram. Nat Med. 2019;25(1):70–4.
93. Gemmell PM, Gillette K, Balaban G, et al. A computational investigation intorate-dependant vectorcardiogram changes due to specific fibrosis patterns in non-ischæmic dilatedcardiomyopathy. Comput Biol Med. 2020;123(103895):103895.
94. Bleijendaal H, Ramos LA, Lopes RR, et al. Computer versus cardiologist: is a machine learning algorithm able to outperform an expert in diagnosing a phospholamban p. Arg14del mutation on the electrocardiogram? Heart Rhythm. 2021;18(1):79–87.
95. Rahman QA, Tereshchenko LG, Kongkatong M, et al. Utilizing ECG-based heartbeat classification for hypertrophic cardiomyopathy identification. IEEE Trans Nanobioscience. 2015;14(5):505–12.
96. Siontis KC, Liu K, Bos JM, et al. Detection of hypertrophic cardiomyopathy by anartificial intelligence electrocardiogram in children and adolescents. Int J Cardiol. 2021;340:42.
97. Grogan M, Lopez-Jimenez F, Cohen-Shelly M, et al. Artificial intelligence-enhanced electrocardiogram for the early detection of cardiac amyloidosis. Mayo Clin Proc. 2021;96:2768.
98. Adam M, Oh SL, Sudarshan VK, et al. Automated characterization of cardiovascular diseases using relative wavelet nonlinear features extracted from ECG signals. Comput Methods Prog Biomed. 2018;161:161(133-43).
99. Zhang X, Walsh R, Whiffin N, et al. Disease-specific variant pathogenicity prediction significantly improves variant interpretation in inherited cardiac conditions. Genet Med. 2021;23:69–79.
100. Quer G, Arnaout R, Henne M, et al. Machine learning and the future of cardiovascular care: JACC state-of-the-art review. J Am Coll Cardiol. 2021;77:300–13.
101. Hermans BJM, Bennis FC, Vink AS, et al. Improving long QT syndrome diagnosis by apolynomial-based T-wave morphology characterization. Heart Rhythm. 2020;17:752–8.

102. Darpo B, Agin M, Kazierad DJ, et al. Man versus machine: is there an optimal method for QT measurements in thorough QT studies? J Clin Pharmacol. 2006;46:598–612.
103. Denny JC, Miller RA, Waitman LR, et al. Identifying QT prolongation from ECG impressionsusing a general-purpose Natural Language Processor. Int J Med Inform. 2009;null:S34–42.
104. Giudicessi JR. Machine learning and rare variant adjudication in type 1 long QT syndrome. Circ Cardiovasc Genet. 2017;10:undefined.
105. Tse G, Chan YWF, Keung W, et al. Electrophysiological mechanisms of long and short QT syndromes. Int J Cardiol Heart Vasc. 2017;14:8–13.
106. Hermans BJM, Stoks J, Bennis FC, et al. Support vector machine-based assessment of theT-wave morphology improves long QT syndrome diagnosis. Europace. 2018;20:113–9.
107. Tse G, Sn L, Zhou J, et al. Territory-wide Chinese cohort of long QT syndrome: random survival Forest and cox analyses. Front Cardiovasc Med. 2021;8:608592.
108. Tse G, Lee S, Li A, et al. Automated electrocardiogram analysis identifies novel predictors of ventricular arrhythmias in Brugada syndrome. Front Cardiovasc Med. 2020;7:618254.
109. Lee S, Zhou J, Li KHC, et al. Territory-wide cohort study of Brugada syndrome in Hongkong: predictors of long-term outcomes using random survival forests and non-negative matrix factorisation. Open Heart. 2021;8(1):e001505.
110. Juhola M, Joutsijoki H, Penttinen K, et al. Detection of genetic cardiac diseases by Catransient profiles using machine learning methods. Sci Rep. 2018;8:9355.
111. Luz EJ, Schwartz WR, Cámara-Chávez G, et al. ECG-based heartbeat classification for arrhythmia detection: a survey. Comput Methods Prog Biomed. 2016;127:144–64.
112. de Chazal P, O'Dwyer M, Reilly RB. Automatic classification of heartbeats using ECG morphology and heartbeat interval features. IEEE Trans Biomed Eng. 2004;51(7):1196–206.
113. de Lannoy G, Francois D, Delbeke J, et al. Weighted conditional random fields for super-vised interpatient heartbeat classification. IEEE Trans Biomed Eng. 2012;59(1):241–7.
114. Zhang Z, Dong J, Luo X, et al. Heartbeat classification using disease-specific feature selection. Comput Biol Med. 2014;46:79–89.
115. Llamedo M, Martinez JP. Heartbeat classification using feature selection driven by data-base generalization criteria. IEEE Trans Biomed Eng. 2011;58(3):616–25.
116. Minhas FU, Arif M. Robust electrocardiogram (ECG) beat classification using discrete wavelet transform. Physiol Meas. 2008;29(5):555–70.
117. Escalona-Morán MA, Soriano MC, Fischer I, et al. Electrocardiogram classification using reservoir computing with logistic regression. IEEE J Biomed Health Inform. 2015;19(3):892–8.
118. Korürek M, Nizam A. A new arrhythmia clustering technique based on Ant Colony Optimization. J Biomed Inform. 2008;41(6):874–81.
119. Luz E, Menotti D. How the choice of samples for building arrhythmia classifiers impact their performances. Annu Int Conf IEEE Eng Med Biol Soc. 2011:4988–91.
120. Mathews SM, Kambhamettu C, Barner KE. A novel application of deep learning for single-lead ECG classification. Comput Biol Med. 2018;99:53–62.
121. Zheng J, Chu H, Struppa D, Zhang J, et al. Optimal multi-stage arrhythmia classification approach. Sci Rep. 2020;10(1):2898.
122. Tomofumi N, Yasutoshi N, Giichi N, et al. Prediction of premature ventricular complex origins using artificial intelligence-enabled algorithms. Cardiovasc Digit Health J. 2021;2:76–83.
123. He K, Nie Z, Zhong G, Yang C, et al. Localization of origins of premature ventricular contraction in the whole ventricle based on machine learning and automatic beat recognition from12-lead ECG. Physiol Meas. 2020;41(5):055007.
124. Zheng J, Fu G, Anderson K, et al. A 12-Lead ECG database to identify origins of idiopathic ventricular arrhythmia containing 334 patients. Sci Data. 2020;23,7(1):98.
125. Zheng J, Fu G, Abudayyeh I, et al. A high-precision machine learning algorithm to classify left and right outflow tract ventricular tachycardia. Front Physiol. 2021;12:641066.
126. Alwan Y, Cvetkovic Z, Curtis MJ. Methods for improved discrimination between ventricular fibrillation and tachycardia. IEEE Trans Biomed Eng. 2018;65(10):2143–51.

127. Mjahad A, Rosado-Muñoz A, Bataller-Mompeán M, et al. Ventricular fibrillation and tachycardia detection from surface ECG using time-frequency representation images as input dataset for machine learning. Comput Methods Prog Biomed. 2017;141:119–27.
128. Picon A, Irusta U, Álvarez-Gila A, et al. Mixed convolutional and long short-term memorynetwork for the detection of lethal ventricular arrhythmia. PLoS One. 2019;14(5):e0216756.
129. Okada DR, Miller J, Chrispin J, et al. Substrate spatial complexity analysis for the prediction of ventricular arrhythmias in patients with ischemic cardiomyopathy. Circ Arrhythm Electrophysiol. 2020;13(4):e007975.
130. Bhattacharya M, Lu DY, Kudchadkar SM, et al. Identifying ventricular arrhythmias and their predictors by applying machine learning methods to electronic health records in patients with hypertrophic cardiomyopathy (HCM-VAr-risk model). Am J Cardiol. 2019;23(10):1681–9.
131. Krittanawong C, Zhang H, Wang Z, et al. Artificial intelligence in precision cardiovascular medicine. J Am Coll Cardiol. 2017;69(21):2657–64.
132. Hu SS, Gao RL, Liu LS, et al. Summary of the 2018 report on cardiovascular diseases in China. Chin Circul J. 2019;2019(3):209–20.
133. Shameer K, Johnson KW, Glicksberg BS, et al. Machine learning in cardiovascular medicine: are we there yet? Heart. 2018;104(14):1156–64.
134. Yancy CW, Jessup M, Bozkurt B, et al. 2013 ACCF/AHA guideline for the Management of Heart Failure. J Am Coll Cardiol. 2013;62(16):e147.
135. Cikes M, Sanchez-Martinez S, Claggett B, et al. Machine learning-based phenogrouping inheart failure to identify responders to cardiac resynchronization therapy. Eur J Heart Fail. 2019;21(1):74–85.
136. Gallard A, Bidaut A, Hubert A, et al. Characterization of responder profiles for cardiac resynchronization therapy through unsupervised clustering of clinical and strain data. J Am Soc Echocardiogr. 2021;34(5):483–93.
137. Galli E, Le Rolle V, Smiseth OA, et al. Importance of systematic right ventricular assessment in cardiac resynchronization therapy candidates: a machine learning approach. J Am Soc Echocardiogr. 2021;34(5):494–502.
138. Kalscheur MM, Kipp RT, Tattersall MC, et al. Machine learning algorithm predicts cardiac resynchronization therapy outcomes: lessons from the Companion trial. Circ Arrhythm Electrophysiol. 2018;11(1):e005499.
139. Feeny AK, Rickard J, Patel D, et al. Machine learning prediction of response to cardiac resynchronization therapy: improvement versus current guidelines. Circ Arrhythm Electrophysiol. 2019;12(7):e007316.
140. Tokodi M, Behon A, Merkel ED, et al. Gender - specific patterns of mortality PredictorsAmong patients undergoing cardiac resynchronization therapy: a machine learning approach. Front Cardiovasc Med. 2021;8:611055.
141. Daubert JP, Zareba W, Cannom DS, et al. Inappropriate implantable cardioverter-defibrillator shocks in MADIT II: frequency, mechanisms, predictors, and survival impact. J AmColl Cardiol. 2008;51(14):1357–65.
142. Milpied P, Dubois R, Roussel P, et al. Arrhythmia discrimination in implantable cardioverter defibrillators using support vector machines applied to a new representation of electrograms. IEEE Trans Biomed Eng. 2011;58(6):1797–803.
143. Mahajan D, Dong Y, Saxon LA, et al. Performance of an automatic arrhythmia classification algorithm: comparison to the ALTITUDE electrophysiologist panel adjudications. Pacing Clin Electrophysiol. 2014;37(7):889–99.
144. Myerburg RJ, Goldberger JJ. Sudden cardiac arrest risk assessment: population science and the individual risk mandate. JAMA Cardiol. 2017;6:689–94.
145. Tsushima T, Al-Kindi S, Nadeem F, et al. Machine learning algorithms for prediction of permanent pacemaker implantation after transcatheter aortic valve replacement. Circ Arrhythm Electrophysiol. 2021;14(3):e008941.
146. Truong VT, Beyerbach D, Mazur W, et al. Machine learning method for predicting pacemaker implantation following transcatheter aortic valve replacement. Pacing Clin Electrophysiol. 2021;44(2):334–40.

147. Sharma PS, Dandamudi G, Naperkowski A, et al. Permanent His-bundle pacing is feasible, safe, and superior to right ventricular pacing in routine clinical practice. Heart Rhythm. 2015;12(2):305–12.
148. Arnold AD, Howard JP, Gopi AA, et al. Discriminating electrocardiographic responses to His-bundle pacing using machine learning. Cardiovasc Digit Health J. 2020;1(1):11–20.
149. Rosier A, Mabo P, Temal L, et al. Personalized and automated remote monitoring of atrial fibrillation. Europace. 2016;18(3):347–52.
150. WHO. WHO cardiovascular diseases (CVDs). n.d. http://www.who.int/mediacentre/fact-sheets/fs317/en/ (accessed February 3, 2018).
151. Lackland DT, Weber MA. Global burden of cardiovascular disease and stroke: hypertension at the core. Can J Cardiol. 2015;31:569–71.
152. Lu J, Lu Y, Wang X, et al. Prevalence, awareness, treatment, and control of hypertension in China: data from 1·7 million adults in a population-based screening study(China PEACE Million Persons Project). Lancet. 2017;390:2549–58.
153. Santos MAGD, et al. Online heart monitoring systems on the internet of health things environments: a survey, a reference model and an outlook. Inform Fusion. 2020;53:222–39.
154. Moraes JL, Rocha MX, Vasconcelos GG, et al. Advances in photopletysmography signal analysis for biomedical applications. Sensors (Basel). 2018;18(6):1894.
155. Ohkubo T, Kikuya M, Metoki H, et al. Prognosis of "masked" hypertension and "white-coat" hypertension detected by 24-h ambulatory blood pressure monitoring 10-year follow-up from the Ohasama study. J Am Coll Cardiol. 2005;46:508–15.
156. Zhang YT, Zheng YL, Lin WH, et al. Challenges and opportunities in cardiovascular health informatics. IEEE Trans Biomed Eng. 2013;60:633–42.
157. Bycroft C, Freeman C, Petkova D, et al. The UK Biobank resource with deep phenotyping and genomic data. Nature. 2018;562:203–9.
158. LeCun Y, Bengio Y, Hinton G. Deep learning. Nature. 2015;521:436–44.
159. Bai W, Sinclair M, Tarroni G, et al. Automated cardiovascular magnetic resonance image analysis with fully convolutional networks. J Cardiovasc Magn Reson. 2018;20:65.
160. Zihlmann M, Perekrestenko D, Tschannen M. Convolutional recurrent neural networks for electrocardiogram classification. Comput Cardiol. 2017;2017:1–4.
161. Lyon A, Mincholé A, Martínez JP, et al. Computational techniques for ECG analysis and interpretation in light of their contribution to medical advances. J R Soc Interface. 2018;15:20170821.
162. Soh DCK, Ng EYK, Jahmunah V, et al. A computational intelligence tool for the detection of hypertension using empirical mode decomposition. Comput Biol Med. 2020;118:103630.
163. Miao F, Wen B, Hu Z, et al. Continuous blood pressure measurement from one-channel electrocardiogram signal using deep-learning techniques. Artif Intell Med. 2020;108:101919.
164. Zhang Y, Zhou C, Huang Z, et al. Study of cuffless blood pressure estimation method based on multiple physiological parameters. Physiol Meas. 2021;42(5):055004.
165. Liu Z, Zhou B, Li Y, et al. Continuous blood pressure estimation from electrocardiogram and photoplethysmogram during arrhythmias. Front Physiol. 2020;11:575407.
166. Li YH, Harfiya LN, Purwandari K, et al. Real-time cuffless continuous blood pressure estimation using deep learning model. Sensors (Basel). 2020;20:5606.
167. Chugh SS, Havmoeller R, Narayanan K, et al. Worldwide epidemiology of atrial fibrillation: a Global Burden of Disease 2010 Study. Circulation. 2014;129(8):837–47.
168. Hannun AY, Rajpurkar P, Haghpanahi M, et al. Cardiologist-level arrhythmia detectionand classification in ambulatory electrocardiograms using a deep neural network. Nat Med. 2019;25(1):65–9.
169. Guo Y, Wang H, Zhang H, et al. Mobile photoplethysmographic technology to detect atrial fibrillation. J Am Coll Cardiol. 2019;74(19):2365–75.
170. Perez MV, Mahaffey KW, Hedlin H, et al. Large-scale assessment of a smartwatch to identify atrial fibrillation. N Engl J Med. 2019;381(20):1909–17.
171. Tison GH, Sanchez JM, Ballinger B, et al. Passive detection of atrial fibrillation using a commercially available smartwatch. JAMA Cardiol. 2018;3(5):409–16.

172. Johnson KW, Torres Soto J, Glicksberg BS, et al. Artificial intelligence in cardiology. J Am Coll Cardiol. 2018;71(23):2668–79.
173. Bai W, Sinclair M, Tarroni G, et al. Automated cardiovascular magnetic resonance imageanalysis with fully convolutional networks. J Cardiovasc Magn Reson. 2018;20(1):65.
174. Bernard O, Lalande A, Zotti C, et al. Deep learning techniques for automatic MRI cardiac multi-structures segmentation and diagnosis: is the problem solved? IEEE Trans Med Imaging. 2018;37(11):2514–25.
175. Jamart K, Xiong Z, Maso Talou GD, et al. Mini review: deep learning for atrial segmentation from late gadolinium-enhanced MRIs. Front Cardiovasc Med. 2020;7:86.
176. Chen HH, Liu CM, Chang SL, et al. Automated extraction of left atrial volumes fromtwo-dimensional computer tomography images using a deep learning technique. Int J Cardiol. 2020;316:272–8.
177. Valinoti M, Fabbri C, Turco D, et al. 3D patient-specific models for left atrium characterization to support ablation in atrial fibrillation patients. Magn Reson Imaging. 2018;45:51–7.
178. Alhusseini MI, Abuzaid F, Rogers AJ, et al. Machine learning to classify intracardiac electrical patterns during atrial fibrillation: machine learning of atrial fibrillation. Circ Arrhythm Electrophysiol. 2020;13(8):e008160.
179. Liu CM, Chang SL, Chen HH, et al. The clinical application of the deep learning technique for predicting trigger origins in patients with paroxysmal atrial fibrillation with catheter ablation. Circ Arrhythm Electrophysiol. 2020;13(11):e008518.
180. Hindricks G, Potpara T, Dagres N, et al. 2020 ESC Guidelines for the diagnosis andmanagement of atrial fibrillation developed in collaboration with the European Association for Cardio-Thoracic Surgery (EACTS): The Task Force for the diagnosis and management of atrial fibrillation of the European Society of Cardiology(ESC) developed with the special contribution of the European Heart Rhythm Association (EHRA) of the ESC. Eur Heart J. 2021;42(5):373–498.
181. January CT, Wann LS, Calkins H, et al. 2019 AHA/ACC/HRS focused update of the 2014 AHA/ACC/HRS Guideline for the Management of Patients with Atrial Fibrillation: A Reportof the American College of Cardiology/American Heart Association Task Force on Clinical Practice Guidelines and the Heart Rhythm Society in collaboration with the Society of Thoracic Surgeons. Circulation. 2019;140(2):e125–51.
182. Inohara T, Shrader P, Pieper K, et al. Association of atrial fibrillation clinical phenotypes with treatment patterns and outcomes: a multicenter registry study. JAMA Cardiol. 2018;3(1):54–63.
183. Ma Z, Wang P, Gao Z, et al. Ensemble of machine learning algorithms using the stackedgeneralization approach to estimate the warfarin dose. PLoS One. 2018;13(10):e0205872.
184. Grossi E, Podda GM, Pugliano M, et al. Prediction of optimal warfarin maintenance dose using advanced artificial neural networks. Pharmacogenomics. 2014;15(1):29–37.
185. Yao X, Abraham NS, Alexander GC, et al. Effect of adherence to oral anticoagulantson risk of stroke and major bleeding among patients with atrial fibrillation. J Am Heart Assoc. 2016;5(2):e003074.
186. Labovitz DL, Shafner L, Reyes Gil M, et al. Using artificial intelligence to reduce theRisk of nonadherence in patients on anticoagulation therapy. Stroke. 2017;48(5):1416–9.
187. Attia ZI, Sugrue A, Asirvatham SJ, et al. Noninvasive assessment of dofetilide plasmaconcentration using a deep learning (neural network) analysis of the surface electrocardiogram: a proof of concept study. PLoS One. 2018;13(8):e0201059.
188. Levy AE, Biswas M, Weber R, et al. Applications of machine learning in decision analysis for dose management for dofetilide. PLoS One. 2019;14(12):e0227324.
189. Iung B, Vahanian A. Epidemiology of valvular heart disease in the adult. Nat Rev Cardiol. 2011;8(3):162–72.
190. Thoenes M, et al. Narrative review of the role of artificial intelligence to improve aorticvalve disease management. J Thorac Dis. 2021;13(1):396–404.
191. Chiang SJ, et al. When and how aortic stenosis is first diagnosed: a single-center observational study. J Cardiol. 2016;68(4):324–8.

192. Cohen-Shelly M, et al. Electrocardiogram screening for aortic valve stenosis using artificial intelligence. Eur Heart J. 2021;42(30):2885–96.
193. Benjamin EJ, et al. Heart Disease and Stroke Statistics-2019 update: a report Fromthe American Heart Association. Circulation. 2019;139(10):e56–e528.
194. Kwon JM, et al. Artificial intelligence for detecting mitral regurgitation using electrocardiography. J Electrocardiol. 2020;59:151–7.
195. Dillon JJ, DeSimone CV, Sapir Y, et al. Noninvasive potassium determination using amathematically processed ECG: proof of concept for a novel "blood-less, blood test". J Electrocardiol. 2015;48(1):12–8.
196. Attia ZI, DeSimone CV, Dillon JJ, et al. Novel bloodless potassium determination using a signal-processed single-lead ECG. J Am Heart Assoc. 2016;5(1):e002746.
197. Lin CS, Lin C, Fang WH, et al. A deep-learning algorithm (ECG12Net) for detecting hypokalemia and hyperkalemia by electrocardiography: algorithm development. JMIR Med Inform. 2020;8(3):e15931.
198. Kwon JM, Jung MS, Kim KH, et al. Artificial intelligence for detecting electrolyte imbalance using electrocardiography. Ann Noninvasive Electrocardiol. 2021;26(3):e12839.
199. Rijnbeek PR, van Herpen G, Bots ML, et al. Normal values of the electrocardiogram forages 16-90 years. J Electrocardiol. 2014;47(6):914–21.
200. Toman O, Hnatkova K, Smetana P, et al. Physiologic heart rate dependency of the PQ interval and its gender differences. Sci Rep. 2020;10(1):2551.
201. Malik M, Hnatkova K, Kowalski D, et al. QT/RR curvatures in healthy subjects: gender differences and covariates. Am J Physiol Heart Circ Physiol. 2013;305(12):H1798–806.
202. Hnatkova K, Toman O, Sisakova M, et al. Gender and race differences in J-Tend, J-Tpeak,and Tpeak-Tend intervals. Sci Rep. 2019;9(1):19880.
203. Ball RL, Feiveson AH, Schlegel TT, et al. Predicting "heart age" using electrocardiography. J Pers Med. 2014;4(1):65–78.
204. Hirota N, Suzuki S, Arita T, et al. Prediction of biological age and all-cause mortality by12-lead electrocardiogram in patients without structural heart disease. BMC Geriatr. 2021;21(1):460.
205. Attia ZI, Friedman PA, Noseworthy PA, et al. Age and gender estimation using artificial intelligence from standard 12-lead ECGs. Circ Arrhythm Electrophysiol. 2019;12(9):e007284.
206. Lima EM, Ribeiro AH, Paixão GMM, et al. Deep neural network-estimated electrocardio-graphic age as a mortality predictor. Nat Commun. 2021;12(1):5117.
207. Strodthoff N, Wagner P, Schaeffter T, et al. Deep learning for ECG analysis: benchmarksand insights from PTB-XL. IEEE J Biomed Health Inform. 2021;25(5):1519–28.
208. Rajput JS, Sharma M, Acharya UR. Hypertension diagnosis index for discrimination of high-risk hypertension ECG signals using optimal orthogonal wavelet filter bank. Int J Environ Res Public Health. 2019;16(21):4068.
209. Sharma M, Rajput JS, Tan RS, et al. Automated detection of hypertension using physiological signals: a review. Int J Environ Res Public Health. 2021;18(11):5838.
210. Ni H, Wang Y, Xu G, et al. Multiscale fine-grained heart rate variability analysis for recognizing the severity of hypertension. Comput Math Methods Med. 2019;2019:4936179.
211. Simjanoska M, Gjoreski M, Gams M, et al. Non-invasive blood pressure estimation from ECG using machine learning techniques. Sensors (Basel). 2018;18(4):1160.
212. Mousavi SS, Hemmati M, Charmi M, et al. Secondary cuff-less blood pressure estimation using only the ECG signal in frequency domain. 2018:147–152.
213. Yang S, Zhang YP, Cho SY, et al. Non-invasive cuff-less blood pressure estimation using a hybrid deep learning model. Opt Quant Electron. 2021;53(2):93.
214. Baker S, Xiang W, Atkinson I. A hybrid neural network for continuous and non-invasiveestimation of blood pressure from raw electrocardiogram and photoplethysmogram waveforms. Comput Methods Prog Biomed. 2021;207:106191.
215. Sagirova Z, Kuznetsova N, Gogiberidze N, et al. Cuffless blood pressure measurement using a smartphone-case based ECG monitor with photoplethysmography in hypertensive patients. Sensors (Basel). 2021;21(10):3525.

216. Laitinen T, Lyyra-Laitinen T, Huopio H, et al. Electrocardiographic alterations during-hyperinsulinemic hypoglycemia in healthy subjects. Ann Noninvasive Electrocardiol. 2008;13(2):97–105.
217. Lipponen JA, Kemppainen J, Karjalainen PA, et al. Dynamic estimation of cardiacrepolarization characteristics during hypoglycemia in healthy and diabetic subjects. Physiol Meas. 2011;32(6):649–60.
218. Ling SH, Nguyen HT. Natural occurrence of nocturnal hypoglycemia detection using hybrid particle swarm optimized fuzzy reasoning model. Artif Intell Med. 2012;55(3):177–84.
219. Phyo Phyo S, Sai Ho L, Nguyen HT. Deep learning framework for detection of hypoglycemic episodes in children with type 1 diabetes. Annu Int Conf IEEE Eng Med Biol Soc. 2016;2016:3503–6.
220. Porumb M, Stranges S, Pescapè A, et al. Precision medicine and artificial intelligence: a pilot study on deep learning for hypoglycemic events detection based on ECG. Sci Rep. 2020;10(1):170.
221. Wang L, Mu Y, Zhao J, et al. IGRNet: a deep learning model for non-invasive, real time diagnosis of prediabetes through electrocardiograms. Sensors (Basel). 2020;20(9):2556.
222. Lin CS, Lee YT, Fang WH, et al. Deep learning algorithm for Management of Diabetes Mellitus via Electrocardiogram-Based Glycated Hemoglobin (ECG-HbA1c): a retrospective cohort study. J Pers Med. 2021;11(8):725.
223. Pham T, Lau ZJ, Chen SHA, et al. Heart rate variability in psychology: a review of HRV indices and an analysis tutorial. Sensors (Basel, Switzerland). 2021;21(12):3998.
224. De Cooman T, Varon C, Hunyadi B, et al. Online automated seizure detection in temporal lobe epilepsy patients using single-lead ECG. Int J Neural Syst. 2017;27(7):1750022.
225. Yamakawa T, Miyajima M, Fujiwara K, et al. Wearable epileptic seizure prediction system with machine-learning-based anomaly detection of heart rate variability. Sensors (Basel). 2020;20(14):3987.
226. Akbilgic O, Kamaleswaran R, Mohammed A, et al. Electrocardiographic changes predate Parkinson's disease onset. Sci Rep. 2020;10(1):11319.
227. Gentili C, Valenza G, Nardelli M, et al. Longitudinal monitoring of heartbeat dynamicspredicts mood changes in bipolar patients: a pilot study. J Affect Disord. 2017;209:30–8.
228. Reinertsen E, Nemati S, Vest AN, et al. Heart rate-based window segmentation improves accuracy of classifying posttraumatic stress disorder using heart rate variability measures. Physiol Meas. 2017;38(6):1061–76.
229. Shah AJ, Lampert R, Goldberg J, et al. Posttraumatic stress disorder and impaired autonomic modulation in male twins. Biol Psychiatry. 2013;73(11):1103–10. https://doi.org/10.1016/j.biopsych.2013.01.019.
230. Frasch MG, Shen C, Wu HT, et al. Brief report: can a composite heart rate variability biomarker shed new insights about autism Spectrum disorder in school-aged children? J Autism Dev Disord. 2021;51(1):346–56.
231. George CF. Diagnostic techniques in obstructive sleep apnea. Prog Cardiovasc Dis. 1999;41(5):355–66.
232. Mendonca F, Mostafa SS, Ravelo-Garcia AG, et al. A review of obstructive sleep apnea detection approaches. IEEE J Biomed Health Inform. 2019;23(2):825–37.
233. Wang X, Cheng M, Wang Y, et al. Obstructive sleep apnea detection using ecg-sensorwith convolutional neural networks. Multimed Tools Appl. 2020;79(23):15813–27.
234. Mashrur FR, Islam MS, Saha DK, et al. SCNN: Scalogram-based convolutional neuralnetwork to detect obstructive sleep apnea using single-lead electrocardiogram signals. Comput Biol Med. 2021;134:104532.
235. Mukherjee D, Dhar K, Schwenker F, et al. Ensemble of deep learning models for sleep apnea detection: an experimental study. Sensors (Basel). 2021;21(16):5425.
236. Morettini M, Peroni C, Sbrollini A, et al. Classification of drug-induced hERG potassium - channel block from electrocardiographic T-wave features using artificial neural networks. Ann Noninvasive Electrocardiol: The Official Journal of the International Society for Holterand Noninvasive Electrocardiology, Inc. 2019;24(6):e12679.

237. Maille B, Wilkin M, Million M, et al. Smartwatch electrocardiogram and artificial intelligence for assessing cardiac-rhythm safety of drug therapy in the COVID-19 pandemic. The QT-logs study. Int J Cardiol. 2021;331:333–9.
238. Johannesen L, Vicente J, Mason JW, et al. Differentiating drug-induced multichannel block on the electrocardiogram: randomized study of dofetilide, quinidine, ranolazine, and verapamil. Clin Pharmacol Ther. 2014;96(5):549–58.
239. Johannesen L, Vicente J, Mason JW, et al. Late sodium current block for drug-inducedlong QT syndrome: results from a prospective clinical trial. Clin Pharmacol Ther. 2016;99(2):214–23.
240. Hoffmann M, Mösbauer K, Hofmann-Winkler H, et al. Chloroquine does not inhibit infection of human lung cells with SARS-CoV-2. Nature. 2020;585(7826):588–90.
241. Chang D-W, Lin C-S, Tsao T-P, et al. Detecting digoxin toxicity by artificial intelligence-assisted electrocardiography. Int J Environ Res Publichealth. 2021;18(7):3839.

# Limitations and Challenges of AI-ECG

# 4

Qing-Peng Zhang, Cheuk To Skylar Chung, Yi-En Li,
Tong Liu, Zhi-Heng Lv, and Jia-Wei Xie

## 4.1 Overview

Qing-Peng Zhang

Cardiovascular and metabolic diseases stand as significant contributors to global mortality. The current approach to assessing electrocardiograms (ECGs) involves a combination of human analysis and automated machine readings. However, these methods are restricted in their ability to extract complex information from ECGs, underscoring the potential for AI advancements to enhance ECG analysis. Novel

Q.-P. Zhang (✉)
Musketeers Foundation Institute of Data Science, The University of Hong Kong,
Pok Fu Lam, Hong Kong, China

Department of Pharmacology and Pharmacy, Li Ka Shing Faculty of Medicine, The
University of Hong Kong, Pok Fu Lam, Hong Kong, China
e-mail: qpzhang@hku.hk

C. T. S. Chung
Cardiac Electrophysiology Unit, Cardiovascular Analytics Group, China-UK Collaboration,
Hong Kong, China

Y.-E. Liu
Queen Elizabeth Hospital, Yau Ma Tei, Hong Kong, China

T. Liu
Department of Cardiology, Second Hospital of Tianjin Medical University, President of
Tianjin Institute of Cardiology, Tianjin, China

Z.-H. Lv
School of Data Science, City University of Hong Kong, Kowloon, Hong Kong, China
e-mail: zhiheng.lyu@my.cityu.edu.hk

J.-W. Xie
The second Hospital of Tianjin Medical University, Tianjin, China

© The Author(s), under exclusive license to Springer Nature Singapore Pte
Ltd. 2024

K.-Y. Chen et al. (eds.), *AI Augmented ECG Technology*,
https://doi.org/10.1007/978-981-97-8359-5_4

algorithms rooted in machine learning and deep learning offer promise in complementing traditional ECG evaluation methods. While recent studies exhibit the feasibility of AI-ECG algorithms for detection, it is vital to acknowledge the distinct challenges and limitations they entail. This chapter aims to cultivate reader understanding and awareness of AI systems, with a focus on addressing present challenges.

As aging populations drive an increased demand for ECGs, the diagnostic potential of this tool remains invaluable for cardiovascular disease diagnosis and evaluation. Yet, the time-intensive nature of ECG interpretation can introduce errors and necessitate significant training efforts [1]. As research burgeons in the realm of AI, its applications in various medical domains, including supervised and unsupervised learning for ECG analysis, are coming to light [2]. Artificial neural networks and support vector machines in supervised learning harness labeled data to learn classification functions, while unsupervised learning leverages unlabeled data for the same purpose [3]. Deep learning, a recent innovation, holds promise in ECG analysis by addressing complex clinical scenarios such as arrhythmia, cardiomyopathy, and heart valve disease, along with non-cardiovascular conditions [4–7]. Unlike conventional machine learning, deep learning adopts an end-to-end approach, deriving essential features directly from raw data and eliminating the need for manually curated feature vectors [8]. This chapter delves into the clinical implications, constraints, and hurdles associated with AI-ECG analysis, enriching our comprehension of this burgeoning field.

## 4.2 Clinical Significance

Zhong Zhuotao and Yi-En Li

Recent investigations underscore the enhanced precision of AI-ECG over conventional ECG software in deciphering rhythm patterns and interpreting ECGs at the onset of cardiovascular symptoms [9]. This capability for immediate risk assessment through AI-ECG holds promise in expediting early identification and preventive measures for vulnerable patients. Notably, AI-powered ECG analysis demonstrates noteworthy accuracy in hypertrophic cardiomyopathy (HCM), yielding a robust AUC of 0.98, along with sensitivities of 92% and specificities of 95% [10]. Machine learning techniques, employed to analyze energy waveform ECGs, effectively pinpoint left ventricular systolic dysfunction [11]. Furthermore, AI-driven ECG analysis proves valuable for gauging risk in close relatives of dilated cardiomyopathy patients [12].

In patients presenting dyspnea in emergency departments, AI-ECG analysis aids in identifying dyspnea stemming from left ventricular systolic dysfunction, surpassing the performance of NT-proBNP [13]. AI also holds the potential to detect unexplained embolic stroke cases that could benefit from oral anticoagulant therapy. Traditional algorithms, in contrast to deep learning algorithms, exhibit diminished reliability in detecting P-waves and extrapolating comprehensive data features concerning atrial fibrillation [14]. However, deep learning algorithms excel in deciphering the intricate signal complexities, fostering a comprehensive understanding of signal parameters [15]. AI-ECG analyses serve as a screening tool for valvular diseases, aiding physicians in identifying moderate to severe aortic stenosis within community settings [16]. In the long term, AI-ECG's potential to provide data-driven clinical decision support for healthcare practitioners is immense.

Beyond cardiovascular disease management, AI-driven ECG data analysis finds applicability in diverse ailments. Deep learning models play a pivotal role in sepsis screening [17]. ECG analysis based on ML identified hyperglycemia with an impressive AUC of 94.5%, coupled with sensitivities of 87.6% and specificities of 85% [18]. This methodology extends to non-invasively assessing physiological parameters, encompassing cardiovascular and cerebrovascular dynamics [19]. By integrating AI-ECG with routine blood chemistry, early diagnosis of recurrent thyroid paralysis becomes feasible while also facilitating the determination of patient ECG age [20].

Recent studies reveal the feasibility and cost-effectiveness of using deep learning models and ECGs to gauge electrolyte imbalances, with wearable devices enabling easy data accessibility [21]. Electrolyte imbalance serves as a pivotal indicator for numerous metabolic disorders, including diabetes insipidus and hyperparathyroidism [22]. Amid the COVID-19 pandemic, AI-ECG analysis attains high negative prediction rates, offering rapid screening to identify healthy individuals [23].

## 4.3 Limitations and Challenges

Tong Liu and Z.-H. Lv

### 4.3.1 Professional Responsibility

Despite the promising potential of AI-ECG, several crucial queries linger at the clinical trial level. The medical domain's obligatory framework for gauging success [24] complicates matters in cases of complications or malpractice, as both human physicians and AI systems are implicated in causality. As AI assumes a larger role in clinical decision-making, it strains the trust dynamics between practitioners and patients. Moreover, an ethical quandary surfaces about determining a physician's professional responsibility in instances of erroneous AI-guided decisions [25]. Additionally, algorithms, prone to random errors, might be unquestionably trusted by inexperienced clinicians. Legal frameworks applicable to contemporary medical products may inadequately address AI liability. Therefore, the development of AI algorithms warrants a level of rigor akin to indications and adverse effect disclosures for other medical products.

### 4.3.2 Discriminatory Bias

AI algorithms often inherit biases from flawed datasets, leading to the specific targeting of certain patient groups. This stems from model bias, arising due to excessive samples of specific types; disparities in models due to underrepresentation of others; and noise resulting from adverse effects of unforeseen variables [26]. Given the variation in ECG characteristics across races, the universal applicability of deep learning algorithms may be compromised [27]. Dependence on electronic data also introduces the risk of data loss or unavailability, potentially causing algorithmic misinterpretation. For instance, specific population groups may have insufficient data available [28]. Furthermore, these systems might misinterpret data due to inadequate healthcare utilization or small sample sizes, wrongly assigning a lower disease burden. Wearable device data could introduce bias toward economically advantaged individuals. Most samples used by university hospital-developed algorithms originate from young, high-income groups in Western countries [28], possibly skewing data interpretation toward a particular subset rather than holistically representing the entire population. This lack of diverse data might exacerbate income disparities. Intriguingly, Noseworthy et al.'s research indicates that even when algorithms are developed using homogeneous populations [27]. Deep learning outcomes are still influenced by race, suggesting an intricate link between algorithmic systems and racial factors.

To address this concern, a potential solution lies in modifying algorithms from a single institution by amalgamating them with data from a more diverse racial and socioeconomic sample. However, this approach necessitates meticulous scrutiny of the sample to ensure its representation across different social strata. Moreover, researchers must be vigilant in identifying any potential discrimination during data analysis.

### 4.3.3 Monitoring and Cybersecurity

The oversight of regulatory government authorities becomes imperative in monitoring the security and precision of specific algorithms. In comparison to other medical products, the vigilance over AI algorithms assumes even greater significance. Upgrades to these systems can potentially impact algorithm performance, underscoring the need to safeguard patients' rights and personal data. The growing anthropomorphism of AI introduces security vulnerabilities and ethical quandaries [29], rendering conventional evaluation methods less effective. Consequently, traditional assessment procedures may be inadequate.

In this context, the emergence of potential security threats looms large, particularly as AI algorithms become targets for malicious intent. The menace of hackers compromising AI algorithms [30, 31] underscores the need for heightened network security. Virtually every facet of the AI architecture, spanning from initial data input to human–machine collaboration and the final data training process, is susceptible to network attacks [29]. Distinct from conventional IT systems, AI systems introduce novel network vulnerabilities [29]. Four primary types of attacks target AI systems [29]: first, attackers can manipulate the classification model to influence the output of the final AI algorithm; second, the AI system's data input can be tainted by false data, considerably decelerating the AI training process; third, through reverse engineering, adversaries can launch multiple adversarial assaults and fabricate counterfeit systems; and finally, adversaries can clandestinely execute backdoor attacks by altering existing classifications and datasets via data contamination.

Recent strides have been made to address these challenges. The US FDA, for instance, has embarked on an ambitious journey toward constructing a stringent regulatory framework for AI's medical applications [32]. In addition, substantial efforts are being invested in safeguarding the e-health sector, exemplified by the development of advanced cyberattack detection systems.

## 4.4 Transformation of Clinical Practice

Qing-Peng Zhang and J.-W. Xie

### 4.4.1 Integration into Clinical Practice

Despite the promising potential of AI in ECG analysis, several specific challenges need to be addressed when implementing AI in clinical settings. While AI medical research often utilizes high-quality ECG datasets and well-defined populations and diseases, real-world scenarios present more complex and heterogeneous challenges. The phenotyping of patient populations is often challenging in clinical practice, leading to disparities in performance between algorithmic results from controlled studies and real-world clinical applications. The variability in ECG data quality further compounds these challenges. Integrating algorithmic findings into the current clinical workflow is another hurdle. While proposed algorithms need rigorous testing and validation, research efforts should also focus on interpreting their results within the context of existing diagnostic tools. Training clinicians to effectively interpret AI-derived information, an often overlooked aspect in research, is essential. With numerous AI-ECG algorithms available, their varied applications for detecting cardiovascular diseases pose challenges in objectively comparing their effectiveness for diverse populations. To bridge this gap, an AI curriculum and training program could equip practitioners with the skills needed to seamlessly integrate AI into clinical practice.

### 4.4.2 Interpretability Challenges

Addressing the lack of interpretability in AI models presents a significant hurdle. Beyond the challenge of comprehending the outcomes generated by operational AI models, further exploration is essential to understand the underlying decision-making mechanisms, a phenomenon commonly referred to as the "black box" problem. To optimize feature representation, researchers often input a multitude of parameters, occasionally numbering in the millions, into AI models [8].

Consequently, researchers are left grappling with the inability to discern the specific features extracted from the 12-lead ECG data utilized by the algorithm [33]. Despite the remarkable performance exhibited by deep learning models, a comprehensive theory explaining their efficacy remains elusive [34]. Within the realm of machine learning, a consensus has yet to emerge regarding the definition of AI explainability [35]. While scientists may comprehend the architecture and fundamental mathematical principles without grasping the complete computational process, this shortcoming diminishes the algorithm's transparency and credibility [34]. This opacity may result in unquantifiable biases that deter clinicians from embracing these algorithms, particularly given the potentially dire consequences of erroneous outcomes. Although interpretability techniques offer some resolution to the challenges posed by the black box problem, their application is not without limitations [36]. Many of these models have only recently emerged and lack rigorous external validation [37]. Presently, the scope of randomized controlled trials for AI systems is restricted [38]. Only by attaining a clear understanding of algorithm interpretability can clinicians identify systemic errors, retrace decision-making processes, and avoid unwarranted reliance. Ongoing research endeavors in algorithm explainability aim to bolster clinician confidence [39]. Notably, overarching frameworks for interpreting AI-ECG classification results have been established, particularly for utilizing 12-lead ECGs [8]. Furthermore, investigations are underway to compare AI-ECG performance with established AF risk-scoring models, including the Heart and Aging Study score in Genomic Epidemiology AF (CHARGE-AF) [37, 40].

### 4.4.3 Logistical Challenges

Machine learning algorithms demand substantial quantities of high-quality data to yield accurate outcomes. This requirement poses a constraint on the development of algorithms applicable to rare disease management, often due to challenges in acquiring sufficient data characterized by incompleteness, heterogeneity, noise, or fuzziness stemming from data loss, redundancy, or sparsity [41]. Multi-center collaborations present a viable solution to this issue. The adoption of standardized data formats, such as Rapid Healthcare Interoperability Resources, could enhance data aggregation [34]. The complexity of existing algorithms, however, impedes their implementation within healthcare institutions due to discrepancies in coding definitions, electronic health record systems, administrative protocols, laboratory equipment, and clinical practices that undermine data generality [38]. These concerns limit the broad adoption of AI models in clinical settings, particularly on portable devices. While compression techniques could mitigate these challenges, they may inadvertently compromise model accuracy. Tailored training specific to individual contexts emerges as a viable avenue for a seamless transition.

## 4.5 Summary

Qing-Peng Zhang

In conclusion, AI-driven ECG analysis is profoundly reshaping diagnostic and prognostic services within both cardiology and non-cardiology realms of the healthcare system. This advancement, while transformative, also ushers in a plethora of novel inquiries encompassing responsibility, technology, and transparency, impacting both medical practitioners and manufacturers. To harness the potential of AI for enhancing healthcare quality, an essential framework governing the integration of AI algorithms must be established. Additionally, researchers must acknowledge the constraints intrinsic to AI-ECG analysis, including potential biases and logistical impediments, and actively engineer interventions to mitigate unfavorable outcomes. By adopting these strategies, the global implementation of AI in clinical practice becomes a tangible reality. Further exploration is now warranted to address any lingering uncertainties inherent in this revolutionary innovation.

## References

1. Bickerton M, Pooler A. Misplaced ECG electrodes and the need for continuing training. Br J Card Nurs. 2019;14(3):123–32.
2. Minchole A, Camps J, Lyon A, et al. Machine learning in the electrocardiogram. J Electrocardiol. 2019;57:S61–4.
3. Krittanawong C, Zhang H, Wang Z, et al. Artificial intelligence in precision cardiovascular medicine. J Am Coll Cardiol. 2017;69(21):2657–64.
4. Lee S, Zhou J, Jeevaratnam K, et al. Paediatric/young versus adult patients with long QTsyndrome. Open Heart. 2021;8(2):e001671.
5. Lima E, Ribeiro AH, Paixão GM, et al. Deep neural network estimated electrocardiographic-age as a mortality predictor. medRxiv. 2021;12(1):5117.
6. Siontis K, Noseworthy PA, Attia ZI, et al. Artificial intelligence-enhanced electrocardiography in cardiovascular disease management. Nat Rev Cardiol. 2021;18(7):465–78.
7. Tse G, Lee S, Zhou J, et al. Territory-wide Chinese cohort of long QT syndrome: random survival Forest and cox analyses. Front Cardiovasc Med. 2021;8:608592.
8. Bodini M, Rivolta MW, Sassi R. Opening the black box: interpretability of machine learning algorithms in electrocardiography. Phil Trans R Soc A. 2021;379(2212):20200253.
9. Kashou A, Mulpuru SK, Deshmukh AJ, et al. An artificial intelligence-enabled ECG algorithm for comprehensive ECG interpretation: can it pass the"Turing test"? Cardiovasc Digit Health J. 2021;2(3):164–70.
10. Siontis K, Liu K, Bos JM, et al. Detection of hypertrophic cardiomyopathy by an artificial intelligence electrocardiogram in children and adolescents. Int J Cardiol. 2021;340:42–7.
11. Potter E, Rodrigues CH, Ascher DB, Abhayaratna WP, Sengupta PP, Marwick TH. Machine learning of ECG waveforms to improve selection for testing for asymptomatic left ventricular dysfunction. JACC Cardiovasc Imaging. 2021;14(10):1904–15.
12. Shrivastava S, Cohen-Shelly M, Attia ZI, et al. Artificial intelligence-enabled electrocardiography to screen patients with dilated cardiomyopathy. Am J Cardiol. 2021;155:121–7.
13. Adedinsewo D, Carter RE, Attia Z, et al. Artificial intelligence-enabled ECG algorithmto identify patients with left ventricular systolic dysfunction presenting to the emergency department with dyspnea. Circ Arrhythm Electrophysiol. 2020;13(8):e008437.

14. Rabinstein A, Yost MD, Faust L, et al. Artificial intelligence-enabled ECG to identify silent atrial fibrillation in embolic stroke of unknown source. J Stroke Cerebrovasc Dis. 2021;30(9):105998.
15. Cardiologs. Real-life application of Artificial Intelligence for ECG analysis. 2021.
16. Cohen-Shelly M, Attia ZI, Friedman PA, et al. Electrocardiogram screening for aorticvalve stenosis using artificial intelligence. Eur Heart J. 2021;42(30):2885–96.
17. Kwon JM, Lee YR, Jung MS, et al. Deep-learning model for screening sepsis using electrocardiography. Scand J Trauma Resusc Emerg Med. 2021;29(1):145.
18. Cordeiro R, Karimian N, Park Y. Hyperglycemia identification using ECG in deep learning era. Sensors. 2021;21(18):6263.
19. Sadrawi M, Lin YT, Lin CH, et al. Non-invasive hemodynamics monitoring system based on electrocardiography via deep convolutional autoencoder. Sensors. 2021;21(18):6264.
20. Lin C, Lin CS, Lee DJ, et al. Artificial intelligence-assisted electrocardiography for early diagnosis of thyrotoxic periodic paralysis. J Endocr Soc. 2021;5(9):bvab120.
21. Kwon J, Jung MS, Kim KHJ, et al. Artificial intelligence for detecting electrolyte imbalance using electrocardiography. Ann Noninvasive Electrocardiol. 2021;26(3):e12839.
22. Papi G, Corsello SM, Pontecorvi A. Clinical concepts on thyroid emergencies. Front Endocrinol. 2014;5:102.
23. Attia Z, Kapa S, Dugan J, et al. Rapid exclusion of COVID infection with the artificial intelligence electrocardiogram. Mayo Clin Proc. 2021;96(8):2081–94.
24. Bazoukis G, Hall J, Loscalzo J, et al. The augmented intelligence in medicine: a framework for successful implementation. Cell Rep Med. 2022;3:n.pag. https://doi.org/10.1016/j.xcrm.2021.100485.
25. Price W, Gerke S, Cohen IG. Potential liability for physicians using artificial intelligence. JAMA. 2019;322(18):1765–6.
26. Barocas S, Selbst AD. Big data's disparate impact. Calif Law Rev. 2016;104:671.
27. Noseworthy P, Attia ZI, Brewer LC, et al. Assessing and mitigating bias in medical artificial intelligence: the effects of race and ethnicity on a deep learning model for ECG analysis. Circ Arrhythm Electrophysiol. 2020;13(3):e007988.
28. Gianfrancesco M, Tamang S, Yazdany J, et al. Potential biases in machine learning algorithms using electronic health record data. JAMA Intern Med. 2018;178(11):1544–7.
29. Lorenzo P, Stefano F, Ferreira A, Carolina P. Artificial intelligenceand cybersecurity: technology, governance and policy challenges. Centre for European Policy Studies (CEPS). 2021; 122 p., 978-94-6138-785-1
30. Muddy Waters Capital LLC. MW is short St. Jude Medical (STJ:US). Muddy Waters Res. 2016;
31. Klonoff D, Han J. The first recall of a diabetes device because of cybersecurity risks. J Diabetes Sci Technol. 2019;13(5):817–20.
32. Food and Drug Administration. Proposed regulatory framework for modifications to artificial intelligence/machine learning (AI/ML)-based software as a medical device (SaMD). 2019.
33. Somani S, Russak AJ, Richter F, Zhao S, Vaid A, Chaudhry F, De Freitas JK, Naik N, Miotto R, Nadkarni GN, Narula J. Deep learning and the electrocardiogram: review of the current state-of-the-art. EP Europace. 2021;23(8):1179–91.
34. Mandel J, Kreda DA, Mandl KD, et al. SMART on FHIR: a standards-based, interoperable apps platform for electronic health records. J Am Med Inform Assoc. 2016;23(5):899–908.
35. Rudin C. Stop explaining black box machine learning models for high stakes decisionsand use interpretable models instead. Nat Mach Intell. 2019;1(5):206–15.
36. Petch J, Di S, Nelson W. Opening the black box: the promise and limitations of explainable machine learning in cardiology. Can J Cardiol. 2022;38(2):204–13.
37. Khurshid S, Friedman S, Reeder C, Di Achille P, Diamant N, Singh P, Harrington LX, Wang X, Al-Alusi MA, Sarma G, Foulkes AS. Electrocardiogram-based deep learning and clinicalrisk factors to predict atrial fibrillation. Circulation. 2021;144(2):122–33.
38. Kelly C, Karthikesalingam A, Suleyman M, Corrado G, King D. Key challenges for delivering clinical impact with artificial intelligence. BMC Med. 2019;17(1):1–9.

39. Doshi-Velez F, Kim B. Towards a rigorous science of interpretable machine learning. arXiv preprint arXiv:1702.08608. 2017.
40. Christopoulos G, Graff-Radford J, Lopez CL, et al. Artificial intelligence-electrocardiography to predict incident atrial fibrillation: a population-based study. Circ Arrhythm Electrophysiol. 2020;13(12):e009355.
41. Griffin F. Artificial intelligence and liability in health care. Health Matrix. 2021;31:65.

# Prospects of AI-ECG

# 5

Zhi-Heng Lv, Lue Tian, Jian-Dong Zhou, and Qing-Peng Zhang

In 1924, Willem Einthoven won the Nobel Prize in Physiology or Medicine for demonstrating that the ECG could detect biological signals from the heart. Since then, ECG has been used as an easily available, low-cost, and non-invasive way to detect cardiac function and diagnose heart disease risk. Since the 1950s, the emergence of analog-to-digital converters has made it possible to process and digitize ECG signals [1], and it has also made it possible to automatically extract, analyze, and interpret ECG signals with the help of computer algorithms [2]. Entering the twenty-first century, with the progress of the times, we have come to the era of big data and AI. At this time, multi-source electronic data came into being, and a variety of large-scale electronic medical record data (such as massive ECG data) appeared in the medical field to record the clinical diagnosis process. These massive ECG data have laid a solid foundation for our technological innovation in the field of data-driven heart disease risk diagnosis. The traditional heart disease analysis methods represented by statistical models are somewhat powerless in today's new situation. With the rapid improvement of hardware computing capabilities represented by graphics processors, AI technology represented by deep learning has ushered in

Z.-H. Lv · L. Tian
School of Data Science, City University of Hong Kong, Kowloon, Hong Kong, China
e-mail: zhiheng.lyu@my.cityu.edu.hk; luetian2-c@my.cityu.edu.hk

J.-D. Zhou
Department of Family Medicine and Primary Care, School of Clinical Medicine, Li Ka Shing Faculty of Medicine, The University of Hong Kong, Pok Fu Lam, Hong Kong, China

Q.-P. Zhang (✉)
Musketeers Foundation Institute of Data Science, The University of Hong Kong, Pok Fu Lam, Hong Kong, China

Department of Pharmacology and Pharmacy, Li Ka Shing Faculty of Medicine, The University of Hong Kong, Pok Fu Lam, Hong Kong, China
e-mail: qpzhang@hku.hk

© The Author(s), under exclusive license to Springer Nature Singapore Pte Ltd. 2024

K.-Y. Chen et al. (eds.), *AI Augmented ECG Technology*, https://doi.org/10.1007/978-981-97-8359-5_5

an era of its own. Compared with the ECG-based heart disease risk diagnosis technology used in the past, the newly applied technology not only improves the accuracy of heart disease risk diagnosis but also creates a series of new application scenarios, including intelligent monitoring based on ECG data, bracelets, etc. What is even more gratifying is that doctors can also use the new data obtained to continuously optimize and update the existing heart disease risk diagnosis model so as to obtain a dynamic disease risk diagnosis and prediction model. Through the analysis of past literature, this chapter believes that the AI technology applied to ECG has the following prospects.

## 5.1 Interpretability Model

Although AI has made great progress in the field of ECG and some deep learning algorithms have high accuracy in predicting certain diseases, the black box characteristics of deep learning still limit its large-scale promotion and application. Most of the deep learning or machine learning currently applied has a black box problem, that is, lack of interpretability. Researchers can use deep learning models to get better results but still cannot understand exactly how today's algorithms perform feature selection [3]. Especially in the medical field, when people are faced with life-or-death decisions, the black box problem of machine learning technology becomes more worrying. Although some machine learning algorithms can predict the results very accurately, because it is difficult for people to understand the logical relationship in the algorithm, even if the effect is good, it is difficult for clinicians to fully trust the final results of the machine learning algorithm [3, 4]. Attia and other researchers [5] explored whether AI and a specific deep neural network can be used to explain the results using artificially selected features when analyzing ECG signals. At the same time, the authors also tried to quantify the interpretability. The model predictions are compared with those manually labeled by experts. The author used canonical correlation analysis to quantify the information of the common features selected by the neural network and humans, respectively, and finally, the author concluded that the features selected by the neural network have a strong correlation with the features selected by experts. In addition, as structured data have gradually attracted the attention of researchers, graphical models have gradually begun to receive attention because of their better interpretability. In future studies, comorbidity networks and patients' electronic health records will include combining ECG data to build interpretable models is a route worth exploring.

## 5.2 Dataset

The datasets used in the current research can be roughly divided into two categories. One is the public datasets such as MIT-BIH. The research using this type of dataset is characterized by high accuracy. It is aimed at a special disease, and the amount of data in the corresponding dataset for the special disease targeted by this kind of research is small, and the trained model often produces overfitting [6–8]. Some studies use unique datasets, and the amount of data extracted and used is relatively sufficient. Still, these studies also have various shortcomings, such as only one medical center, and the problem of multiple medical centers in different regions is insufficiently explored [9]. Insufficient datasets and insufficient data volume make the obtained results unable to be used to verify whether it is feasible for different regions [4, 10]. However, due to the small dataset, the obtained results cannot prove whether using model labeling will be better than manual labeling results. For the research of some wearable devices, the data provided by wearable devices is too noisy, which brings great difficulties to the training model [11]. At the same time, machine learning also has biases in the selection of datasets, such as researchers' biases in sampling and selecting datasets [3]. Therefore, higher-quality datasets are still needed in future research.

## 5.3 Clinical Trial Verification

Although AI technology provides us with a new method for predicting certain diseases, there is a mature framework for the evaluation of predictive models, and all models, including AI models, must follow this framework. Any prediction model needs to have accurate prediction results, as well as prospective clinical trials in a large-scale heterogeneous population and improvement in clinical diagnosis results so that the model can be proved to be clinically feasible. In order to test the predictive ability of the model, both discrimination and calibration need to be tested at the same time. The current AI research often focuses on evaluating the model using the discriminant matrix while often ignoring the calibration ability of the model. Calibration power, which reflects how closely a model approximates the predicted probability of an event to the observed frequency of events, is assessed by plotting the actual observed event frequency against the average predicted probability for each decile of the sample. For clinical practice, a reliable model requires both good discrimination and proper calibration [12]. For some wearable devices, the research must be carried out in a real environment to know whether the algorithm used is suitable. In short, since real clinical practice is much more complicated than the experimental simulation, even if the deep neural network can obtain the results more accurately in the experimental situation, the researchers still need to carry out rigorous and a large number of experiments to verify whether the obtained algorithm is real or not reliable. For example, in a study conducted by researchers at the Mayo Clinic, a deep neural network was used to distinguish patients with hyperkalemia. Although the accuracy of AUC was 0.853, the final result was relatively low in specificity. There are 42% false positive results in the obtained results, and these may bring unnecessary tension and inconvenience to patients in clinical practice. There may be many reasons for false positives, and this requires re-exploration and optimization of existing problems in rigorous experiments [13].

## 5.4 Manual Marking Method

The inaccuracy of manual labeling will affect the results obtained by machine learning algorithms [14]. For some diseases below the diagnostic criteria, such as amyloidosis [15], due to the particularity of this disease, there may also be undiscovered diseases in the control group, so the inaccuracy of artificial markers will also affect the obtained results. In the case that manual marking cannot improve higher accuracy, we can use the method of combining ECG data with other data to improve the accuracy of the model, such as the collaborative application of ECG and intracardiac electrical recording, imaging technology, etc. to improve the risk stratification accuracy of patients [16]; or combine ECG with other biological knowledge and data to improve the performance of the model [17]. For different but similar diseases, the lack of accurate labels prevents researchers from obtaining classification results for more diseases. At the same time, most of the current research is focused only on the diagnosis of a certain type of disease, and the labeling of ECG in the manual labeling process is limited only to a certain disease, so the obtained AI model can judge only a certain disease. There are still many limitations in clinical practice, and it is also a future research direction to train algorithms that can comprehensively judge the problems existing in patients' ECG and even give diagnosis and treatment recommendations [18].

## 5.5 Assist Doctors and Help Patients

Looking forward to the future, depending on the application scenario, the new technologies required will be different, but it is important for researchers to clarify that the purpose of the constructed model is not to replace doctors but to assist doctors or patients (Fig. 5.1). In terms of assisting doctors, it can be applied to disease prevention [19, 20], disease diagnosis and treatment [18, 21–23], and prognosis management, such as an article published on *Nature Communications*, Lima [24] will use a deep learning network to process ECG. The post-predicted age data are

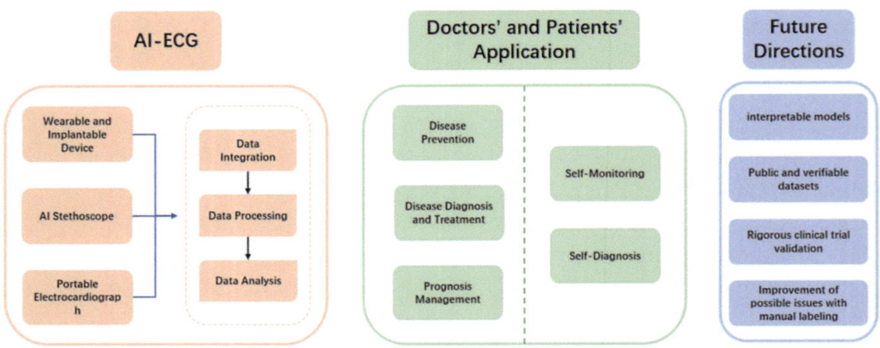


**Fig. 5.1** Application and future direction of AI-ECG

compared with the actual age of the patient, proving that ECG can be used to assist doctors in predicting mortality and provide additional prognostic information. For patients, it can be applied to self-test and self-diagnosis [25–27].

For specific application scenarios such as wearable devices, the ECG data that these portable instruments can provide is significantly different from the data that can be measured in traditional hospitals and can provide long-term ECG data (providing data anytime and anywhere, such as providing the wearer's ECG data at different time periods of the day), rather than short-term, so through the same mapping method to obtain ECG data, portable devices can provide long-term ECG data with more information, so AI based on richer information algorithms will also perform better. However, at present, the ECG generated by wearable devices such as smartwatches is obtained by a single-lead or multi-lead method, while the ECG recorder in the hospital is often obtained by the 12-lead ECG data, and the 12-lead ECG data contains more information, which can better describe the electrical signal activity of the heart, which is, therefore, more conducive to the application of AI methods. In order to allow portable devices to play a greater role in the field of personal health management, it is very promising to develop a new generation of ECG recording devices with more effective mapping methods, such as textiles embedded with sensors, while considering comfort and safety [28]. ECG data often contains errors (noise) generated during the measurement process (equipment accuracy, measurement operations, etc.), so more accurate equipment is needed to obtain ECG data, and more effective noise reduction algorithms and models are needed to extract more accurate data from the ECG signal [29].

At the same time, for specific diseases, according to an article published in *Nature Reviews Cardiology*, the future application of AI-ECG can be summarized into the following aspects [30].

- Atrial Fibrillation: Going beyond the CHA2DS2-VASc score to combine ECG marker risk of stroke with electronic health record-based clinical information, imaging, and biomarkers; rhythm pattern recognition utilizing implantable and wearable cardiovascular electronics to predict atrial fibrillation events; use AI-enhanced ECG to guide patients with paroxysmal atrial fibrillation to use "pocket pills," such as guiding patients to take oral anticoagulants or IC antiarrhythmic drugs; smartphone-based QT interval monitoring for patients who start or take long-term sotalol, dofetilide, or other drugs that may affect initial repolarization.
- Sudden Cardiac Death: Determining which patients should be implanted with an ICD can be combined with clinical data and imaging markers.
- Predict the worsening of congestive heart failure based on continuous ECG ambulatory data, thereby preventing emergency room visits and hospitalizations.
- To judge and stage the severity of patients with heart failure, heart valve disease, and pulmonary artery disease and to assist doctors in making clinical decisions, prognosis, and monitoring of hypertensive patients.

- For angina and stress ECG analysis, to assist physicians in selecting high-risk patients who would benefit from invasive arterial assessment and possible intervention.

As an important part of precision medicine, digital twins can not only be used for auxiliary diagnosis, auxiliary treatment, and prognosis assessment but also in the fields of clinical trials and medical equipment test upgrades [31]. Thanks to the rapid development of communication technology, the exchange of information between various devices has become more convenient, so it is also possible to build a personalized digital twin by using computers to analyze massive amounts of personal data. Information obtained from different devices, including personal data information, personal physiological and pathological information (gene sequence, gene expression level, and personal health status), living environment, living habits, etc., can be used to train machine learning models [32–34]. After the data are obtained, a personalized digital twin is constructed by combining the physical model and the machine learning model [31]. By analyzing various data of patients, the personalized digital twin can reflect the real health status of patients in real time, which helps doctors diagnose diseases. For example, left ventricular myocardium stiffness and attenuated diastolic activity tension can be assessed by fitting a physical model to diastolic pressure data and images [35, 36], or they can be assessed using simulations on a digital twin before the patient receives treatment. The effect of the therapy is to help doctors identify a treatment that is more suitable for the patient's actual situation. For improving ablation guidance in cases of myocardial infarction with ventricular tachycardia, the patient's digital twin can assist doctors in locating the specific condition of the patient before the clinical operation, enabling the identification of the best target [37]. With the help of the patient's digital twin, before the clinical operation, the doctor can locate the specificity of the patient and identify the best target. Digital twins can also be used to assess the risk of patient prognosis and provide guidance and assistance to patients in their daily lives. For example, digital twin doctors are used to conduct risk assessments on patients with hypertrophic cardiomyopathy and give corresponding suggestions to patients with different risk levels when participating in certain sports, thereby reducing the risk of sudden death due to exercise [38]. Digital twins can also participate in product development, and the simulation results obtained can be used to supplement nonclinical trials, that is, to introduce virtual patients to enhance clinical trials. For example, the US FDA accepted the use of computer simulation results as an alternative to preclinical animal testing in the study of artificial pancreas control strategies [39]. ECG signals, as a description of an individual's cardiac health, are an important component of a personalized digital twin. With the continuous development of digital twin technology, ECG data will play an important role in the fields of precision medicine and scientific research with the popularization of digital twins.

## 5.6 Summary and Outlook

Although AI technology applied in the medical field is still relatively new compared to other fields such as image recognition, speech recognition, and word processing, the progress of AI technology in the medical field still receives a lot of attention. AI applied in the field of ECG is in the ascendant, and we are witnessing a brand new era of AI-ECG. Recent AI-ECG technology demonstrates the potential of using machine learning to improve detection accuracy and confidence, which could ultimately help physicians improve the quality of clinical diagnosis and access to high-quality medical care. At the same time, advances in hardware have also helped us start thinking about how to reshape the patient's diagnosis and treatment process. Although these technologies still have shortcomings, we believe that in terms of AI algorithms applied to ECG, researchers can improve the problems of manual labeling by solving the interpretability of the model and providing high-quality verifiable datasets. After review, inspection, verification, and strict training for doctors, AI-ECG will be more hopeful to change the field of clinical diagnosis and treatment and bring great help to both doctors and patients. Looking to the future, we are pleased to see that AI-ECG has a bright future.

## References

1. Taback L, et al. Digital recording of electrocardiographic data for analysis by a digitalcomputer. IRE Trans Med Electron. 1959;3:167–71.
2. Caceres CA, et al. Computer extraction of electrocardiographic parameters. Circulation. 1962;25(2):356–62.
3. Somani S, et al. Deep learning and the electrocardiogram: review of the currentstate-of-the-art. EP Europace. 2021;23(8):1179–91.
4. Ko W-Y, et al. Detection of hypertrophic cardiomyopathy using a convolutional neuralnetwork-enabled electrocardiogram. J Am Coll Cardiol. 2020;75(7):722–33.
5. Attia ZI, Lerman G, et al. Deep neural networks learn by using human-selected electrocardiogram features and novel features. Eur Heart J Digit Health. 2021;2(3):446–55.
6. Jahmunah V, et al. Automated detection of coronary artery disease, myocardial infarction and congestive heart failure using Gabor CNN model with ECG signals. Comput Biol Med. 2021;134:104457.
7. Chiou Y-A, Hung C-L, et al. AI-assisted echocardiographic prescreening of heart failure with preserved ejection fraction on the basis of Intrabeat dynamics. JACC Cardiovasc Imaging. 2021;14(11):2091–104.
8. Fu L, et al. Hybrid network with attention mechanism for detection and location of myocardial infarction based on 12-lead electrocardiogram signals. Sensors. 2020;20(4):1020.
9. Kwon JM, et al. Artificial intelligence for detecting electrolyte imbalance using electrocardiography. Ann Noninvasive Electrocardiol. 2021;26(3):e12839.
10. Ware P, et al. Implementation and evaluation of a smartphone-based telemonitoring program for patients with heart failure: mixed-methods study protocol. JMIR Res Protocol. 2018;7(5):e121.
11. Bax JJ, van der Bijl P, et al. Machine learning for electrocardiographic diagnosis of left ventricular early diastolic dysfunction. J Am Coll Cardiol. 2018;71(15):1661–2.
12. Liu Y, et al. How to read articles that use machine learning: users'guides to the medical literature. JAMA. 2019;322(18):1806–16.

13. Galloway CD, et al. Development and validation of a deep-learning model to screen forhyperkalemia from the electrocardiogram. JAMA Cardiol. 2019;4(5):428–36.
14. Hannun AY, et al. Cardiologist-level arrhythmia detection and classification in ambulatory electrocardiograms using a deep neural network[J]. Nat Med. 2019;25(1):65–9.
15. Goto S, et al. Artificial intelligence-enabled fully automated detection of cardiac amyloidosis using electrocardiograms and echocardiograms. Nat Commun. 2021;12(1):1–12.
16. Miao F, et al. Continuous blood pressure measurement from one-channel electrocardiogramsignal using deep-learning techniques. Artif Intell Med. 2020;108:101919.
17. Zhang Y, et al. Study of cuffless blood pressure estimation method based on multiplephysiological parameters. Physiol Meas. 2021;42(5):055004.
18. Lih OS, et al. Comprehensive electrocardiographic diagnosis based on deep learning. Artif Intell Med. 2020;103:101789.
19. Al-Zaiti S, et al. Machine learning-based prediction of acute coronary syndrome usingonly the pre-hospital 12-lead electrocardiogram. Nat Commun. 2020;11(1):1–10.
20. Avanzato R, Beritelli F. Automatic ECG diagnosis using convolutional neural network. Electronics. 2020;9(6):951.
21. Lee S, et al. Temporal variability in electrocardiographic indices in subjects with Brugada patterns. Front Physiol. 2020;11:953.
22. Tse G, et al. Automated electrocardiogram analysis identifies novel predictors of ventricular arrhythmias in Brugada syndrome. Front Cardiovasc Med. 2021;7:399.
23. Tse G, et al. Incorporating latent variables using nonnegative matrix factorization improves risk stratification in Brugada syndrome. J Am Heart Assoc. 2020;9(22):e012714.
24. Lima EM, et al. Deep neural network-estimated electrocardiographic age as a mortalitypredictor. Nat Commun. 2021;12(1):5117.
25. Soh DCK, et al. A computational intelligence tool for the detection of hypertension using empirical mode decomposition. Comput Biol Med. 2020;118:103630.
26. Marston HR, et al. Mobile self-monitoring ECG devices to diagnose arrhythmia that coincide with palpitations: a scoping review. Healthcare (Basel). 2019;7(3):96.
27. Reading M, et al. Factors influencing sustained engagement with ECG self-monitoring: perspectives from patients and health care providers. Appl Clin Inform. 2018;9(4):772–81.
28. Tripathi PM, et al. A review on computational methods for Denoising and detecting ECG signals to detect cardiovascular diseases. Arch Comput Method Eng. 2021;29:1–40.
29. Nigusse AB, Mengisite DA, Malengier B, et al. Wearable smart textiles for long-term electrocardiography monitoring —a review. Sensors. 2021;21(12):4174.
30. Siontis KC, et al. Artificial intelligence-enhanced electrocardiography in cardiovasculardisease management. Nat Rev Cardiol. 2021;18(7):465–78.
31. Corral-Acero J, Margara F, Marciniak M, et al. The "digital twin" to enable the visionof precision cardiology. Eur Heart J. 2020;41(48):4556–64.
32. Khoury MJ. Precision medicine vs preventive medicine. JAMA. 2019;321(4):406.
33. Noble D. Evolution beyond Neo-Darwinism: a new conceptual framework. J Exp Biol. 2015;218(1):7–13.
34. Lamata P. Teaching cardiovascular medicine to machines. Cardiovasc Res. 2018;114(8):e62–4.
35. Xi J, Lamata P, Niederer S, et al. The estimation of patient-specific cardiac diastolicfunctions from clinical measurements. Med Image Anal. 2013;17(2):133–46.
36. Wang ZJ, Wang VY, Bradley CP, et al. Left ventricular diastolic myocardial stiffnessand end-diastolic myofibre stress in human heart failure using personalised biomechanical analysis. J Cardiovasc Transl Res. 2018;11(4):346–56.
37. Prakosa A, Arevalo HJ, Deng D, et al. Personalized virtual-heart technology for guidingthe ablation of infarct-related ventricular tachycardia. Nat Biomed Eng. 2018;2(10):732–40.
38. Lyon A, Ariga R, Mincholé A, et al. Distinct ECG phenotypes identified in hypertrophiccardiomyopathy using machine learning associate with arrhythmic risk markers. Front Physiol. 2018;9:213.
39. Kovatchev BP, Breton M, Dalla Man C, et al. In silico preclinical trials: a proof of concept in closed-loop control of type 1 diabetes. J Diabetes Sci Technol. 2009;3(1):44–55.

MIX
Papier aus verantwortungsvollen Quellen
Paper from responsible sources
FSC® C105338

If you have any concerns about our products,
you can contact us on
**ProductSafety@springernature.com**

In case Publisher is established outside the EU,
the EU authorized representative is:
**Springer Nature Customer Service Center GmbH**
**Europaplatz 3, 69115 Heidelberg, Germany**

Printed by Libri Plureos GmbH
in Hamburg, Germany